The Hamptons Diet
Cookbook

Also by Fred Pescatore, M.D.

The Hamptons Diet
The Allergy and Asthma Cure
Thin For Good
Feed Your Kids Well

The Hamptons Diet Cookbook

Enjoy the Hamptons Lifestyle Wherever You Live

Fred Pescatore, M.D.
and
Jeff Harter

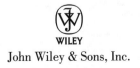

John Wiley & Sons, Inc.

Published by John Wiley & Sons, Inc., Hoboken, New Jersey
Published simultaneously in Canada

Design and composition by Navta Associates, Inc.

Insert credits: Photographs by Joseph Deleo. Prop styling by Bill Samios. Food styling by Anthony Leberto.

For general information about our other products and services, please contact our Customer Care Department within the United States at (800) 762-2974, outside the United States at (317) 572-3993 or fax (317) 572-4002.

Wiley also publishes its books in a variety of electronic formats. Some content that appears in print may not be available in electronic books. For more information about Wiley products, visit our web site at www.wiley.com.

Library of Congress Cataloging-in-Publication Data:

Pescatore, Fred, date.
  The Hamptons diet cookbook : enjoy the Hamptons lifestyle wherever you live / Fred Pescatore and Jeff Harter.
      p. cm.
  Includes bibliographical references and index.
    ISBN-13 978-0-471-79215-4 (cloth)
    ISBN-10 0-471-79215-2 (cloth)
  1. Weight loss. 2. Diet. I. Harter, Jeff. II. Title.
RM222.2.P47 2006
641.5'635—dc22

                                                                            2006006460

Printed in the United States of America

10   9   8   7   6   5   4   3   2   1

To SHF, without whom I could accomplish nothing.
Now I am a complete person.

—*Fred Pescatore*

To my son, Diego.

—*Jeff Harter*

CONTENTS

FOREWORD

I have been cooking for a long time and very rarely does something come along that changes the way I've been doing things—the Hamptons Diet did just that. I now live in Chicago where I am a celebrity chef and a best-selling cookbook author. However, before Chicago, I was a private chef in East Hampton.

One day when I was appearing on a television show in Chicago, I met Dr. Fred. I was on the show to promote Common Threads, a nonprofit organization that seeks to create a sanctuary for children to embrace diversity and cultural differences. Dr. Fred was there to promote his book *The Hamptons Diet*. Upon hearing about the Hamptons Diet, my ears perked up and I listened to what the man had to say.

He spoke about things that I cherish—whole foods, eating from the bounty of the earth, and trying to be in harmony with our surroundings—and, of course, the food he was making on camera smelled delicious and looked sublime in its simplicity.

Dr. Fred was cooking with an ingredient I had barely heard of: macadamia nut oil. He gave me a bottle to cook with and since that day, I have not been able to put it down. It has literally changed my cooking life, and, of course, changed the palates of those I cook for.

Macadamia nut oil has a wonderful, light buttery flavor that is great in both cold and hot dishes. The subtle flavor is great on everything from fish to desserts, and it does not lose its flavor when heated. The oil got me for those reasons; but, as Dr. Fred explained, the oil is incredibly healthy and good for us—what could be better?

I also have been interested in cooking healthy foods that taste good. Dr. Fred and the Hamptons Diet really take us back to basics. The thought of using clean food that is local to your area, fresh from farm stands (or as close as you can get it), and eating foods that are in season may sound like a novel idea, but it is something that has been going on for centuries that was lost only recently.

Dr. Fred and the Hamptons Diet impressed me because everything I used to do when I worked in the Hamptons Dr. Fred was espousing in his book. I used to go to the same vegetable stands, shop at the same farms for meats, and I really learned to follow the changing seasons of the year with the meals I created. I never felt so healthy as when I was eating and preparing foods in this way.

We all want a lot of variety and not to get bored when we are eating. Cooking the Hamptons Diet way teaches us how to never get bored. By learning a few recipes where the ingredients can easily be swapped out, by having a few kitchen essentials, and by knowing how to pick the proper foods, you can create a lasting gift of health for you and your family.

Dr. Fred has prepared us to lead a whole life. By teaching us to eat and cook with whole foods and whole grains, and enjoy fresh fruits and vegetables again, Dr. Fred is taking us to the future by revisiting the past. This fresh and wholesome approach has changed the way I cook and I know it will change the way you cook, too. Please enjoy, and happy eating.

—Art Smith, author of *Back to the Table*

ACKNOWLEDGMENTS

I would like to acknowledge my patients, staff, friends, and family for the inspiration to spread this message of health.

—Fred Pescatore, M.D.

I would like to acknowledge my mother and father for teaching me how to eat well at a young age, Cheryl for her support and enthusiasm, Alison for hiring me over the Internet, and Fred for giving me this great opportunity.

—Jeff Harter

The Hamptons Diet Cookbook

Introduction

Welcome to the Hamptons! To me, the Hamptons are more a state of mind than an actual place. With the success of my previous book, *The Hamptons Diet*, I made many appearances around the country to promote this wholesome eating plan. One of the most oft-repeated questions I heard was, why the Hamptons? To those of you who haven't read the original book, I'll explain some of the premises behind the diet. I had the notion that in order to motivate people to lose weight and get healthy, the food actually had to taste good, even to the point that the dieter felt a little self-indulgent. Yet the diet also needed to produce results and really get those pounds to budge. Because I wanted the diet to be healthy—no fads, no gimmicks, just good old-fashioned ideas that have stood the test of time—I searched the literature to see which diets were based on sound scientific data.

The most credible one was the Mediterranean diet. This type of eating plan has been proven for a hundred or more years to lower cholesterol and decrease the risk for developing all other cardiovascular diseases—plus, the food tastes good. When I asked people what they knew about the Mediterranean diet, though, they all said the same thing—pizza and pasta. Those of you who have been fortunate enough to make a trip to Italy, Spain, Turkey, or Greece, to name a few countries where this type of cooking is prominent, know that there is so much more to Mediterranean cooking than these two dishes. So, I had to change people's perception of what the Mediterranean style of cooking is, as well as update it and make it healthier along the way. The result was the Hamptons Diet.

My cookbook coauthor, Jeff Harter, has a long tradition of working with the Mediterranean lifestyle—he spent ten years cooking in Spain. I was lucky to have found him when a good friend of mine, the local restaurateuse Alison Becker Hurt, introduced us. She is the proprietor of a restaurant named Alison, currently in Bridgehampton; it has been a mainstay of the East End restaurant scene for many years. She also ran Alison on Dominick Street in New York City.

The Hamptons Diet was about to hit the bookstores, and I was searching for someplace to host the book release party when Alison mentioned that she was reopening in a new space and had just hired a new chef whom she had brought over from Spain. When I went to the opening and saw the menu, I couldn't believe my eyes. The food on that menu could have been lifted directly from my book, and I hadn't even met this chef yet.

I asked the chef, Jeff Harter, to cater the launch party for my book. It was an overwhelming success, and our partnership was formed. Because *The Hamptons Diet* had become a best-seller, I wanted to have a companion cookbook so that people could take full advantage of eating healthier. When the offer came from the publisher, I had only one person in mind to help with the recipes—Chef Jeff. This book's recipes are mostly his creations, with inspiration from me, his girlfriend, my patients, and, of course, the Hamptons. While Jeff is my coauthor and has contributed many of the recipes, the text was written by me—Dr. Fred—in my voice.

Jeff is originally from Boulder, Colorado. After attending college in San Diego, he worked in various restaurants, learning the trade on the job. Jeff had a passion for Mediterranean cuisine and felt that he needed actual cultural experience to advance his knowledge of the cuisine. He set off for

Spain. There, he spent time in the kitchens of several very famous restaurants: Candido in Segovia, one of the most well-known and respected restaurants in Spain, which is more than a hundred years old; El Bulli in Rosas, a three-star Michelin restaurant, where he worked under Ferran Adria; and Arzak in San Sebastian, also a three-star Michelin restaurant. After a brief stint in Manhattan at Il Buco restaurant, Jeff headed for the Hamptons and took an executive chef position at Alison in Bridgehampton, where he presents his Basque country–influenced cuisine—a perfect complement to the *Hamptons Diet*.

The Hamptons Diet Cookbook is a new concept. It's one of the first cookbooks to be written by both a chef and a doctor—what a great way to make a diet healthy! My love affair with food started as an infant. If you've read any of my books, you know that I was an overweight child, adolescent, and young adult. I have spent the rest of my years learning how to lose weight and get healthy. I love food. Both of my parents were great cooks, and they taught me everything I know: how to shop for the freshest ingredients, how to choose ripe fruits and vegetables, never to keep food in the house for too long, to eat seasonally and locally, and how to cook for large groups. You know how certain Italian American families cook—as if there is no tomorrow. The one thing I had to teach myself was the art of cooking just enough, and that has been the hardest lesson to learn.

I started cooking in medical school, and the older I got, the more practiced I became. You can trace my level of cooking sophistication by following the recipes in my books. For the most part, I created every recipe in each book—except for this one. With the success of *The Hamptons Diet*, I got to meet chefs all over the country and the world, and many of them wanted to send me their interpretations of healthy Hamptons cuisine. I'm thrilled to share some of these recipes with you in this book. Many of my patients and Hamptonites who have visited my Web site have also contributed recipes. I love getting everyone involved. Cooking and eating healthy can be fun, quick, and easy, and that's the most important lesson to learn from this book.

The recipes range from complicated and taxing, for the serious food network–addicted cooks out there, to quick and easy solutions to the age-old question "What's for dinner?" Most recipes can be made in less than thirty minutes—shorter than the time needed to pick something up, order in, or heat a frozen packaged dinner. Preparation is the key to success in the kitchen. This book will show you the shortcuts that a chef uses, as well as those used by a working person who likes to cook.

People of most dieting persuasions will be tempted by the recipes in this book. Those of you on any diet ranging from Atkins to the Zone will be able to find recipes to suit your dietary needs. *The Hamptons Diet Cookbook* is primarily for individuals who want to be healthy—the weight loss is an added bonus.

If you are interested in the latest trend of slow-release carbohydrates, you won't be disappointed. The recipes include many healthful slow-release carbohydrates and are balanced according to the glycemic index and the glycemic load, naturally. That's the beauty of eating the Hamptons Diet way. I have taken the guesswork out of how to be healthy. There is no need to count calories, carbohydrates, fat, or anything else.

The Hamptons lifestyle is all about eating food that's fresh, local, and organic, if possible. *The Hamptons Diet Cookbook* shows you how to make it taste delicious. Please enjoy.

~ 1 ~

The Hamptons Diet
Principles

The Hamptons Diet is one of the first diet programs designed around the concept of slow-release carbohydrates. For the last twelve years, I have recommended eating healthy carbohydrates. The main problem with the low-carbohydrate movement was that people couldn't get beyond thinking that the only way to lose weight was to eliminate all carbohydrates and stick solely to proteins. I have always advocated eating healthy carbohydrates, which are now termed *slow carbs*. The Hamptons Diet concept is to make balanced moderation sexy.

The Hamptons Diet is a Mediterranean diet that I've updated to reflect how Americans eat today; it also includes an entirely new ingredient— macadamia nut oil. I was so impressed with macadamia nut oil as a healthful cooking ingredient that I formed a company to import it into the United States because it was relatively scarce when I first began to talk about it. Recently, many people have started to use the oil, and it is now commonly available throughout this country and the world.

This chapter of the book is for anyone who has not read *The Hamptons Diet* or who follows a different eating program and has bought this book for its delicious recipes. The next few pages explain the basic principles of the Hamptons eating lifestyle.

The Hamptons Diet— It's as Easy as A, B, or C

There are three phases to the Hamptons Diet. Each recipe in the book specifies which phase of the diet that dish is suited for. Jeff and I tried to make most of the dishes fit every phase of the diet. Only a few are just for the advanced stages of the diet program. Since I can't explain the complete diet in this cookbook, simply use the following pyramids as a guide, or read *The Hamptons Diet* for the full explanation.

The A plan is for people who are just starting on their weight-loss regimen. It's the most restrictive phase of the program; however, you'll soon discover that it's not that restrictive at all. There are many delicious, satisfying recipes for you to eat. Follow this program if you want to lose weight.

The B plan is for people who have no weight to lose or else they are trying to learn to eat more healthfully. This is the transition phase of the program. You have lost weight on the A plan and are now within five pounds of your goal; therefore, you need to learn how to incorporate more foods into your eating regimen and continue at this level.

The C plan is for people who have finished losing weight or have learned to avoid obviously unhealthful foods and are looking for a lifestyle approach to weight management and wholesome eating.

Rebuilding the Food Pyramids

To help you understand the many complexities of the food chain and how it translates into healthy eating, I devised a method using tools that most of us are somewhat familiar with—food pyramids. Because even the new and improved USDA food pyramid isn't very user-friendly, I broke up the categories of food into their various components: proteins, carbohydrates (vegetables, grains, and fruits), and fats.

By using these pyramids, you can easily figure out how to eat in any situation. My patients have even photocopied the pyramids, shrunk these to wallet- or purse-size, laminated them, and now carry the pyramids wherever they go. If they get hungry or are in a restaurant or a grocery store, they check the pyramid to see where a particular food falls, and if it's on the bottom tier, they know it's safe and healthy to eat.

Since each pyramid has a slightly different set of rules, I'll explain them individually.

The Protein Pyramid

Generally, all foods in this category are permitted; however, it is healthier to limit the top two tiers of foods because they either have more calories or are more highly processed. That's not to say that you should avoid those foods entirely, as some of my recipes incorporate each of these foods, but you should do your best to limit them. Eggs are a perfectly acceptable form of protein, and you are encouraged to eat them. The old wives' tale about eggs raising one's cholesterol needs to be banished. If you buy organic eggs,

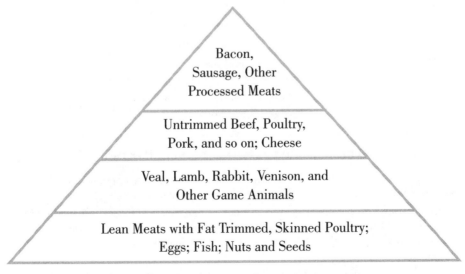

Bacon,
Sausage, Other
Processed Meats

Untrimmed Beef, Poultry,
Pork, and so on; Cheese

Veal, Lamb, Rabbit, Venison, and
Other Game Animals

Lean Meats with Fat Trimmed, Skinned Poultry;
Eggs; Fish; Nuts and Seeds

THE PROTEIN PYRAMID

they are one of Mother Nature's most perfect foods and are also a natural cholesterol-lowering agent. Don't be afraid to enjoy them.

The Carbohydrate (Vegetable) Pyramid

For this pyramid, avoid the top tier when you are trying to lose weight and eat most of your vegetables from the bottom tier. This applies to the dieters using the A program from the book.

If you are on the B program, which is for people who need to lose only a few pounds or you have already lost as much as you want to and are making the transition to a new, healthier lifestyle, you are free to choose from the bottom two tiers.

Individuals on the C, or maintenance, program are free to choose from any of the tiers of the pyramid. Keep in mind, though, that vegetables on the top tier are quite starchy and should be held to a minimum.

Since so many vegetables are available, here is a simple rule: if a vegetable is not listed in the top or the bottom tier, it can be placed in the middle tier.

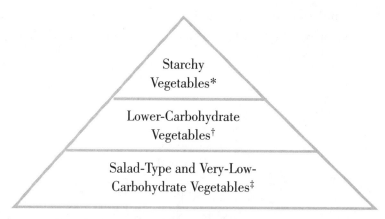

Starchy
Vegetables*

Lower-Carbohydrate
Vegetables†

Salad-Type and Very-Low-
Carbohydrate Vegetables‡

THE CARBOHYDRATE (VEGETABLE) PYRAMID

*Starchy vegetables are peas, cooked carrots, corn, potatoes, winter squash (butternut, buttercup, etc.), beets, parsnips, jicama, breadfruit, cassava, plantains, and christophene.

†Lower-carbohydrate vegetables include eggplant, onion, tomato (although technically a fruit), broccoli, cauliflower, asparagus, cabbage, leeks, scallions, water chestnuts, zucchini, string beans, avocados, spaghetti squash, turnips, artichoke hearts, okra, collard greens, and dandelion greens.

‡Salad vegetables include lettuces of all types, spinach, kale, fennel, mushrooms, bok choy, celery, radishes, peppers, bean sprouts, and cucumbers.

The Carbohydrate (Grain) Pyramid

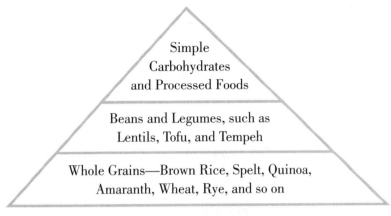

Simple
Carbohydrates
and Processed Foods

Beans and Legumes, such as
Lentils, Tofu, and Tempeh

Whole Grains—Brown Rice, Spelt, Quinoa,
Amaranth, Wheat, Rye, and so on

THE CARBOHYDRATE (GRAIN) PYRAMID

The top tier should be avoided as much as is humanly possible, though, of course, we are all going to have birthdays and special occasions to celebrate. For people trying to lose weight, the foods on the bottom tier are permitted in a ½-cup serving three times per week while on the A program, up to five days per week on the B program, and foods from the bottom two tiers are permitted every day on the C program.

Some of the grains you see on the pyramid may be unfamiliar to you, but if you want to lead a healthy lifestyle, you'll learn to love them. They are generally tastier than the average grain and pack a lot more nutrients into a meal. Spelt, amaranth, quinoa, kamut, teff, and other odd-sounding whole grains are readily obtainable in many mainstream supermarkets and are certainly available in natural food stores. Please be adventurous. In this book and in *The Hamptons Diet*, you will find recipes that teach you how to use these grains. The main difference is in the cooking time. They tend to need more cooking, unless they are in the form of pasta, in which case they'll need less cooking—the more al dente, the better.

The Fruit Pyramid

The bottom tier is for people on the A program. Individuals on the B plan can indulge in the fruits listed on the bottom two tiers, and those on C may

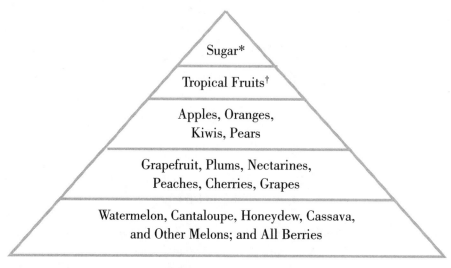

THE FRUIT PYRAMID

*Sugar includes but is not limited to corn syrup, high-fructose corn syrup, beet sugar, maple syrup, fructose, sucrose, cane sugar, brown rice syrup, honey, and most things that end in -ose and -ol.

†Tropical fruits include bananas, pineapples, guavas, mangos, papayas, passionfruit, and so on.

indulge in the bottom three tiers. Tropical fruits are the highest in sugar and should be avoided almost all the time, unless you are on an exotic tropical vacation. In fact, the average banana contains six teaspoons of sugar. Sugar must be avoided at all times, but beware, as it comes in many disguised forms.

The Fat and Oil Pyramid

This is a crucial pyramid and the one that influences health the most. For optimal health, choose only the oils from the bottom tier of this pyramid and avoid all others when you can control the situation. Obviously, when you're out and about, you won't always know what oil is being used. Simply assume the worst, because you will probably be right. Even if the restaurant is using olive oil, it is more than likely using the cheapest brand it could find, which almost universally means that the oil has been processed.

If you take a moment to study the pyramids, you will have more than enough information to change your eating habits for the better. For a more complete list of foods, I refer you to *The Hamptons Diet*.

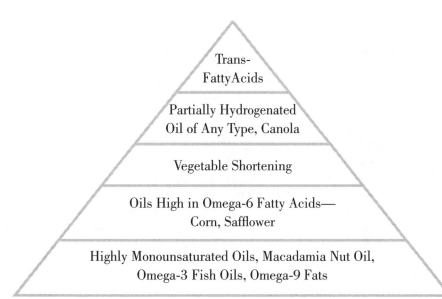

THE FAT AND OIL PYRAMID

Hamptons Diet Acceptable and Unacceptable Foods at a Glance		
Food Type	*Eat*	*Don't Eat*
Proteins	Lean meats with the fat trimmed and the skin removed	Untrimmed meats, too much bacon/sausage or milk
Fish/Omega-3 fats	Most fish, including salmon, trout, sardines, halibut, northern tuna—buy from tested, protected waters, wild only; flaxseeds	Fried and breaded fish
Fruits and Vegetables	Lots of vegetables and low-sugar fruits	High-sugar tropical fruits like bananas; limit corn, peas, potatoes, and tomatoes (really a fruit)
Beans, Legumes, and Nuts	Macadamia, Brazil, walnut, pecan, lentils, and beans	Honey-roasted nuts, peas; try to limit peanuts
Grains	Whole grains only—the word *whole* must appear on the *ingredient* list, not just on the label.	White foods: pasta, rice, biscuits, pretzels, refined carbohydrates, and processed, prepackaged foods

(continued)

Hamptons Diet Acceptable and Unacceptable Foods at a Glance (*continued*)

Food Type	Eat	Don't Eat
Oils	Macadamia nut oil—second choice is avocado oil, estate-bottled extra-virgin olive oil for cold uses	Every other oil, including any types of spreads or margarine
Fats	Monounsaturated-rich sources; emphasis on whole foods and *no* trans-fatty acids	No fried food, chips, crackers, packaged or processed foods; read labels to avoid anything that is hydrogenated or partially hydrogenated
Alcohol	5 oz. of wine; 1½ oz. of distilled spirits	Limit to two servings for women and four servings for men per week
Dairy	Cheese, butter/ghee, heavy cream	Margarine, milk (of any fat content), ice cream, yogurt/kefir (except for C-level dieters)

To make this even easier for people who aren't familiar with the program, here are the Hamptons Diet top ten rules.

1. Use macadamia nut oil as your main cooking oil; avocado oil as your second choice; estate-bottled olive oil for cold uses, such as salad dressings.

2. Avoid sugar.

3. Avoid trans-fatty acids, which are found primarily in packaged and processed foods, including that classic American fare, fast food. Be careful with the new labeling laws and all of the packaged foods proclaiming that they're without trans fats—the label can say zero trans fats even if the serving contains 0.5 grams. That may seem trivial, but if you consume three servings twice a day of a food product like that, and given the minuscule serving sizes of packaged foods, you will have gotten 3 grams of trans fats—enough to increase your risk

for cardiovascular disease if consumed on a regular basis. This section includes margarine, spreads, and shortenings.

4. Avoid simple carbohydrates—nothing white, including pretzels, bagels, breads, pasta, and rice.

5. Avoid oils that are high in omega-6 fatty acids—corn, sunflower, safflower, soybean, peanut, grapeseed, and highly processed oils, such as canola and most olive oils.

6. Incorporate more fatty fish into your diet, but please buy only wild and from sources that test their catch for mercury and PCBs.

7. Eat nuts, legumes, and beans in moderation and as snacks.

8. Eat only *whole* grains—the word must appear in the ingredient list.

9. Eat large amounts of vegetables, and limit fruits to those that contain the least amount of sugar.

10. Drink moderate amounts of alcohol, as outlined previously.

2

A Healthy Kitchen Equals Healthy Food

It's obvious that I believe the foundation for healthier eating comes from healthier foods, but food is only part of the equation. Where your meals are prepared is just as important as the ingredients themselves. The cooking oils you choose are another vital step, and learning how to shop in a healthy way is the final piece of the puzzle. Once you master those four steps, the rest is easy. I'll teach you everything you need to know.

The Kitchen

I'm a doctor, so let's start with a "physical" of your kitchen. Kitchens come in all shapes and sizes, just like my patients. With the correct care, though, they can all be healthy. In this section, I won't ask that you bring in a bulldozer and start from scratch. I just want to show you that with a few insights and ideas, you can upgrade the health of your cooking space, even though you may not be able to afford that remodeling you've been dreaming about.

Whether you have a hot plate with one pot and one pan or a full cook's kitchen, by following some of my tips and suggestions, it can be the perfect setting for you to create delicious, wholesome, and healthy meals for you and your family.

One of the most delicious and healthy meals I have ever enjoyed in my travels through kitchens around the world was in the American West on an organic beef ranch. The meal was prepared by a cowboy chef at his chuck wagon. Along with the few essential pieces of cutlery and wooden spoons he had on hand, all the chef used to complete the meal was a skillet, a dutch oven, and a beautiful well-seasoned wooden salad bowl. With this spare array of equipment and one burner—his campfire—he prepared an outstanding meal of organic beef stew, complete with local root vegetables and a wonderful salad. I must admit, the peach cobbler dessert smelled great, but I promise, I did not partake.

With any "physical," we must first assess the state of the patient. So hold onto your book, grab a pad and a pencil, and let's go to your kitchen.

Pots, Pans, and Even Your Grandmother's Cast-Iron Skillet

This section is really not about suggesting brands of cookware. That is an individual decision based on economics. In a perfect kitchen, however, you should use ceramic-covered aluminum cookware—now can you guess my favorite brand? This allows for even cooking throughout the pots and the pans. My second-favorite choice is copper pots and pans. They look great and do a dynamite job. Any pots and pans will do, though, if you have the right ones. For this reason, I also won't recommend how many saucepans and skillets you should own, but I will say the more the merrier. A true cook, however, can use one pot to make a great meal. Many of the recipes in this book and in my previous books can be made with just one pot or pan.

No matter which brand you own, if you use nonstick skillets or pots, please choose the type where the nonstick coating doesn't eventually become unstuck from the utensil and end up in your food. Older finishes like Teflon tend to eventually flake off the surface of the pan. Yuck—and certainly not healthy.

Another thing I would steer clear of are your old aluminum pots and pans. Put them in the garage, the basement, or the attic—anywhere but the kitchen. The newer brands of aluminum pots and pans are probably fine because they are tempered so that the aluminum doesn't leach into the food. Stainless steel tends to make foods sticky and does not heat evenly, so I tend to avoid it.

I actually still have and use my grandmother's cast-iron skillet. A correctly seasoned cast-iron pot or skillet is a great utensil to have when preparing fish, fowl, meat, or even vegetables. Cast-iron cookware helps on many levels. The nature of the cast iron and its ability to perform well at high heat help us to prepare foods quickly, which keeps more of the vitamins and the nutrients in the food. Also, it is the original nonstick cookware. This means that when grilling and sautéing, you won't need to have your food swimming in oil. Oil can be healthy, but let's not go overboard. Oil is not a sauce.

Baking Items

+ Heavy stainless-steel baking sheets and roasting pans, not flimsy aluminum, are preferred.

+ Heat-resistant glass and ceramic, high-quality metal, and any of the enamel-coated metal casseroles work fine for oven use.

+ Watch out for the nonstick baking sheets and muffin pans. If you do use them, please work with the newer versions where the nonstick surface won't eventually flake off into your food.

Please note that I'm not trying to dictate how you should stock your kitchen—a million other cookbooks and Martha Stewart can provide that information. I simply want to teach you how to tweak what you may already have to make yours the healthiest kitchen on the block.

Cutting Boards

The improper use of cutting boards can be a source of cross-contamination. Cross-contamination means mixing raw meat or poultry juices with cooked food or contaminating cooked food with the juices of raw foods. This is easily done while transporting food to the oven or removing it from the grill, but it happens most frequently during the preparation of food.

To avoid this, have at least three cutting boards on hand.

- ✦ Use a nonabsorbent cutting board for poultry, fish, and meat. It's much easier to ensure that you get all of the bacteria off the surface when the board is nonabsorbent. There are great heavy-duty plastic boards available that can even go directly into the dishwasher.

- ✦ Use a wooden cutting board for all your veggies.

- ✦ Finally, I like to have an extra smaller wooden cutting board around for those you-never-know-when-you-may-need-one moments.

For example, friends are visiting for dinner, I'm using one wooden cutting board to prepare my fennel salad, and someone wants a lemon or a lime wedge to put in his mineral water or martini. Problem solved. Here's the lime. Here's the board. Here's the paring knife. Now go to the bar and let me finish cooking!

Having several cutting boards ensures a smooth flow in the kitchen. When you have a smooth flow, things go more quickly and everything takes less time.

When handling perishable foods, please clean your hands with an anti-bacterial soap and dry them on a paper towel that you can discard before you touch any of the other foods you prepare for that meal. Remember, too, that even though dish towels are pretty, they can hold and spread bacteria until you wash them. Sponges also can easily spread bacteria, so make sure they are clean and rinsed when you take them from one food prep area to another. If you choose to rinse off poultry or any meat or fish item, be careful of where the water splashes—it will also carry bacteria. When it comes to protein foods that will be cooked thoroughly, there is really no health reason to clean them with water, because any potential contaminant will be destroyed by the heat.

Appliances

An efficient kitchen should be equipped with all the usual suspects—blender, food processor, handheld mixer, and so on—but I do have a few other suggestions that I find quite useful.

- An electric hand-held immersion blender is a wonderful gadget that comes in handy when you want to quickly blend ingredients directly in the pot without having to remove them to a mixing bowl. It's also a great way to finish off a gravy, a sauce, or a dressing with fresh herbs, to add that extra brightness and depth of flavor just before you drizzle the sauce on one of your delicious creations.

- Another appliance I find essential in my kitchen is a mini-food processor. I use mine almost every day. It's an easy way to chop and mince perfectly if you don't have the expertise of a chef who does this by hand. Mini-food processors are wonderful for grating hard cheeses and mixing organic herbs—both fresh and dried—to make delicious, unique combinations. These little wonders are amazing time savers.

Utensils

Most of us have drawers full of utensils: knives, wooden spoons, tongs, spatulas, wire whisks, and so on. My old adage holds true here—the more things you have, the easier and the faster cooking becomes. Without the right tools, you can't build anything—the same holds true for cooking. You wouldn't try to chop down a tree with a pair of scissors! Of course, you can have a healthy kitchen without having a spoon for every occasion—but after all, a spoon is not just a spoon. So here are my suggestions for this category:

- Take a few minutes and put all of your utensils on the countertop. Weed out the ones you don't use that often—wooden spoons with cracks in them, plastic spoons that have seen better days, and those rubber spatulas that have somehow gotten burned—and either throw them away or relegate them to the back of the drawer. They will only get in the way, thus increasing the time necessary to complete the meal, or else they have been compromised and the elements of the utensils—plastic, rubber, wood—are seeping into your food.

- Regarding rubber spatulas, which are quite handy, don't use them when you need to mix something over the flame. Heat affects the rubber, and it can melt into your food.

Mixing Bowls, Measuring Cups, and Storage Containers

It's important to always have enough mixing bowls and storage containers on hand. This allows for easy preparation and also lets you save food for the rest of the week, for lunches, and so on. I am a big fan of leftovers. They're incredibly versatile, and I couldn't live without them. Often, I'll prepare meals on Sundays or Mondays because I'm not in the office on those days. Then I just reheat these dishes on other days when I'm much too busy to cook. This works especially well for breakfast and lunch. I'll make a huge frittata and then munch on it for the rest of the week—it's great even as a snack. Here are my suggestions for this category:

- The healthiest choice of materials for mixing bowls and storage containers include metal, glazed ceramic, and glass instead of plastic. I am concerned that the chemicals in plastic can leach into the food.

- Measuring cups and spoons are crucial for two reasons. First, they help us follow the recipe and stay on track as the ingredients in a dish work together to create the final product. Furthermore, if you don't know why a certain ingredient is in a recipe, you may change the dish by changing the amount of that ingredient. Second, I admit that adding ingredients by feel is part of any chef's repertoire, but sometimes we tend to get carried away, and extra calories don't need to find their way into a dish.

- Throw away anything that has any chips or cracks, because it may affect the contents of what it will hold. Just get rid of the offending item, and buy a new one.

- Always use paper bags, not plastic, to store refrigerated produce.

- When freezing items, use freezer paper or glass containers.

- Avoid aluminum foil or plastic wrap. My rule of thumb is *whatever touches food becomes part of the food.*

Miscellaneous Must-Haves

There are a few items in my kitchen that I find very useful and consider my must-haves. Having certain tools allows you the freedom and flexibility to prepare great dishes that you can't do with ordinary kitchen tools. You may have some of these items already. If so, great; if not, they are definitely worth investing in.

- *Meat Thermometer.* These are really useful tools. Because oven temperatures vary, so will cooking times. Therefore, a good-quality meat thermometer becomes your independent register of when your food is correctly cooked because you can read the food's interior temperature. When you have the benefit of these inexpensive kitchen tools, you'll never undercook, which with some foods holds health risks. You will never overcook either, which guarantees that you will maintain the maximum vitamin and nutrient content of whatever you prepare.

- *Mandolin.* This is the missing link between knives and the slicing attachment on a food processor. This implement makes it easier to slice thinly and uniformly, without having the expertise of a chef and without the mess of a food processor. You can find mandolins available in a wide range of prices, with many blade attachments. Whichever you choose, the function is the same. My only suggestion is that you are confident in the sharpness of the blade.

   This tool will be essential when you follow some of our creative "ravioli" recipes. To be able to slice ultra thinly not only heightens the visual aesthetics of the finished product, but it gives you the freedom to serve certain foods raw that you may have had to blanch or steam to serve before. This allows you to prepare meals that have maximum vitamin and nutrient value because nothing has been lost during cooking. Imagine snacking on wafer-thin slices of raw organic fennel and parmesan cheese drizzled with lemon-infused macadamia nut oil and fresh cracked pepper while you peruse the recipes in this book to find just the perfect dinner for tonight.

- *Vegetable Brush.* When you are buying organic vegetables, especially in little local markets, they still have dirt or sand on them. A vegetable brush makes it easier to clean them. Also, if you are grilling, these brushes allow you to paint the marinade on really easily with a minimum of mess to you or the grill.

+ *Wood File.* Believe it or not, a carpenter's wood rasp is a phenomenal grating tool in the kitchen for certain hard things.

During a medical school break, I traveled to Italy to the towns where my grandparents were born. I was invited to the home of a family whose members were friends of my grandfather on my father's side. Naturally, it was dinnertime, and, of course, the meal followed the tradition of all Italian families. Many courses. One of these courses was pasta. Back then, my feelings about flour were not as they are today, so, of course, I ate what was put in front of me. It was a beautiful plate of delicate pumpkin ravioli in a simple butter sauce.

When my plate was placed on the table, Mama took out a carpenter's rasp and grated a touch of nutmeg on top. Before I knew it, there was quite a lively discussion between Mama and Papa. I really didn't understand the words themselves, but I concluded that Papa had been looking for his rasp for days and couldn't figure out how it had disappeared from his wood shop.

Conclusion—Carpenter's rasps are good. Not pilfering them from the pegboard in the garage is better.

+ *Butcher's Twine.* Besides its obvious use for meats and poultry preparation, butcher's twine comes in handy when you have a bunch of fresh organic herbs that you won't completely use for your meal. Simply tie them at the base, and hang them until they are dry. Presto—homemade dried organic herbs that can last for months.

+ *Cutlery Shears.* These scissorlike snippers that usually come with your cutlery set actually have a use. For instance, when you are fileting your wild fish, they are great for snipping off the fins. Another time they come in handy is when you cook artichokes; the shears make it simple to cut the pointy tips from the leaves before you steam them.

+ *Zesting Rasp.* Many foods are taken to a whole new level if you add a bit of citrus zest just before serving them. This also increases the amount of vitamin C and citrus bioflavonoids (which you get only through the supplementation of citrus rinds) in the dish.

- ✦ *Vegetable Steamer.* Simply put, when you steam your vegetables above boiling water instead of boiling them in the water, they retain more of their vitamin and nutrients.

- ✦ *RealSalt.* This is a particular brand of salt that I think is the best salt on the market. It's mined from an ancient sea bed in the mountains of Utah. It's filled with minerals and makes foods taste sensational. Whenever the recipes call for salt, try to make it RealSalt.

- ✦ *MacNut Oil.* Again, this is my company and a brand choice. It's the best macadamia nut oil on the market today. It's unprocessed, and the oil isn't exposed to heat at any time during the crushing of the nuts. It is superior to the other brands and is available in many stores or online, if not in a store near you. To spray pans with macadamia nut oil, buy a spray bottle specifically made for this use from a kitchen store. Fill the bottle with oil, and keep the bottle handy for when you need a light coating of oil.

- ✦ *Salad Spinner.* This is one of my favorite kitchen items. You should always wash any produce or fresh herbs that you buy, especially the organic ones. Rinse the items under water and let the spinner do all the work.

Under the Sink

A healthy kitchen doesn't stop with the food and the tools. You can buy many kitchen cleaning supplies that have minimal impact on the environment. I suggest that you start looking for them. Each region of this country has different ones, so I won't name brands. Suffice it to say that taking care of the environment plays a big role in our health.

Healthy Ingredients

I told myself I wouldn't resort to the old line "You are what you eat," but I couldn't restrain myself. No truer words have ever been spoken, and so many people don't understand that simple concept. When it comes right down to it, our bodies are nothing more than machines, and if we don't get the proper fuel, we don't function properly. It always amazes me that people who would never consider putting leaded or low-octane fuel in their cars don't think twice about stuffing their faces with doughnuts. If you want peak performance, go for peak ingredients.

The Hamptons Diet eating philosophy can be summed up quite succinctly: fresh, local, seasonal, and organic, if possible.

If you stick to those few buzzwords when shopping, you will always have healthy ingredients. Of course, it isn't possible to eat this way all the time—for example, in the dead of winter—but it is how our ancestors ate, and they were usually not overweight. All fruits and vegetables have growing seasons in every part of the world. There are summer and winter foods. With the advent of free trade and airplane journeys, it's possible to eat any food you want at any time of the year, but all research is pointing to the fact that this isn't the healthiest way to eat. Apples are a winter fruit, and grapes are a summer fruit. Zucchini is a summer vegetable, and butternut squash is a winter vegetable.

The Thanksgiving meal is the closest to a seasonal meal that most of us ever get. The Pilgrims ate what was available at that time of the year—thanks to the Native Americans. That's what I mean by eating seasonally and locally. Since America is so big and has so many different climates, each of us will have different foods available throughout the year, so it's impossible for me to tell you exactly what to eat.

I learned to eat this way because that's what the Hamptons symbolize to me. They're not all about movie stars, bankers, and mansions. The farms still exist, at least for now. I'm able to go to the beach and catch my dinner. I can drive or walk to a nearby farm stand and get delectable fresh, local, and seasonal fruits and vegetables, and, lucky for me, they are organic, too. If I have to choose between locally grown and organic, though, I always choose local. They taste better and have the vitamins, the nutrients, and the minerals we need to best sustain us.

I don't always have the opportunity to be in the Hamptons, and many of you who read this won't be shopping there either, but in many major cities, rural towns, and suburbs, there is ample opportunity to get farm-fresh food. New York City has greenmarkets where the fresh abundance of the Hudson

Valley is brought down to us city folk. One can also join an organic growing co-op, where fresh, local, organic, and seasonal fruits and vegetables are delivered directly to one's door each week. They are even less expensive than the grocery stores, at least in New York City. I urge you to find those services in your area. I would bet they are there, and you've just never noticed. If you can't find or can't afford any of these things, that's okay, too. Just pick the fruits and the vegetables that are seasonal in your climate—that's better than nothing.

Healthy Shopping Tips

+ *Learn Your Grocery Store.* This is the biggest obstacle with my patients. If you are like me, you know exactly where everything is in the grocery store where you usually shop. This makes for an easy in and out. I'm asking you now, though, to look for different foods with funny names, and you may have no idea where to find them. This takes more time, and we all hate to waste time on such things, don't we? So, I suggest that you take a morning and do this without the kids and the spouse. Look at what is on the shelves. Go down aisles that you normally whiz by. Once you do this a couple of times, locating the healthier foods becomes just as routine as shopping for all of your old unhealthy foods. It is a small investment to make on the road to health.

+ *Shop the Perimeter.* Most grocery stores keep the fresh foods along the perimeter of the store. The outside aisles have fruits and vegetables, leading to the back of the store, which is dairy and meats, then up the other side of the store, which has deli and freezer sections and more dairy, usually. That's where you are apt to find the healthier food selections—fresh, seasonal, and often organic, too. The inner aisles of the store are where packaged and canned foods are located—try to avoid these as much as possible.

+ *Buy Extra.* When at a farm stand or even the local grocery store, if you see great produce and fruits, buy more than you need. If you refrigerate them, it will slow down their aging process and they'll last longer. Also, you can make vegetable and fruit purees that can be frozen for the leaner months.

✦ When fresh herbs are on sale or they look especially fresh and good, buy extra. These can be hung upside down and dried or chopped in a mini-food processor or a blender, and you will have great organic herbs through the winter.

✦ In my healthy kitchen, you will always find herbs and spices (these can make any meal unique); cans of wild, mercury-free salmon and tuna (great for a quick meal, even breakfast); and various soup stocks in the freezer (these are simple to make on a snowy or rainy day from organic meat bones that are available at the butcher's for practically nothing).

I also just go to the grocery store every day and get what looks fresh.

Keep in mind that what goes on a food label is determined by lobbyists, lawyers, and food manufacturers, not people who are necessarily interested in your health. The only place to find out exactly what is in the product is to look at the ingredient list—never believe the label.

The best example of this is "whole wheat bread." When you go to a deli or a diner and ask for whole wheat bread, you are almost always getting brown white bread, not whole wheat. If you don't believe me, go to the store and look at a common popular brand of wheat bread, not one of the good ones. The word *whole* may not appear in the ingredient list—if it doesn't, you aren't getting a whole-grain bread.

I will translate a few of the most common buzzwords so that you won't be fooled when you go shopping.

Breaking the Code

✦ *Organic.* This is probably the biggest, most contentious issue right now. There are currently no federal guidelines on the definition of "organic." There are state guidelines, but most of them are pretty flimsy. The guidelines are different for animal and vegetable sources. In my opinion, *organic* should mean that for fruits and vegetables, the soil hasn't received any man-made fertilizer for at least five years, the seeds used to grow the foods weren't genetically modified, and the plants weren't sprayed with chemicals of any kind. Sounds pretty reasonable, but this usually does not happen. As for animals, they should eat the diet they would naturally have in the wild. For cows and sheep, this is grass. For poultry, it is earthworms, grasshoppers, and other insects picked off the ground. For fish, it is other fish, algae, plankton, and the like. I am unsure what the natural food for pigs is, so I can't comment on that. Feeding the animal anything other than its natural diet changes the fatty acid profile in its flesh, making it less healthy and beneficial for us to consume. Also, the land on which animals graze or live should not have been chemically fertilized. There are other considerations as well. You can see how difficult it is to get truly organic foods.

- *Non-GMO*. This means the crop has been grown without the use of genetically engineered seeds. The major chemical companies have developed seeds that grow into plants that will not die if serious and dangerous chemicals are used on them to kill pests. This is being done with America's two biggest crops—corn and soybeans. When you consider that corn is almost ubiquitous in our society, we are part of this great unmonitored experiment. These crops were never tested in human safety studies. In fact, on one of the genetically modified corn species, the butterfly that pollinates the plant dies when it tries to pollinate this genetically modified corn. If it can do that to a butterfly, what is it doing to our health? Europeans are much more aware of this than we are and have tried to stop the imposition of these crops in their countries; most of them have been successful. The Third World countries, however, have not been as successful in banning these seeds, and since so much of our food is produced in these countries, we must be very diligent. Look for "Non-GMO" on the label.

- *Free Range*. This is used to describe the conditions in which the poultry live. It generally means the birds are able to run around, get exercise, and act somewhat like normal animals; however, there is no regulation as to how many animals are kept in one place, what they are fed, or how many hours they are allowed to run free. While this is probably better than the conditions that typical commercial hens are kept in, it's hard to determine the exact health benefits we get from poultry or eggs that are just free range if the carton doesn't also specify hormone-, antibiotic-, and pesticide-free, as well as list the type of feed (for example, "they were not fed any animal by-products").

◆ *No Sugar Added*. As you may be aware, there are at least thirty-five different substances to sweeten a product with that technically aren't sugar—barley malt, brown rice syrup, fructose, sucrose, and so on. At least sugar is a natural product that grows in soil, and if grown organically, it is probably a better sweetener than others.

◆ *Hormone Free*. This means that the animal was not given growth hormones. Why we give our animals growth hormones is beyond me. This is more an issue with beef than with other meats. The original thought was so that the animal would produce more milk, yet we have a glut of milk and have to dump millions of gallons each year. Again, this is a huge subsidy that the American government gives to the pharmaceutical companies. Look for hormone-free foods. I think part of the reason why obesity is so rampant is due to the growth hormone residue found in the foods we consume.

◆ *Natural*. This term has no real definition. The most common usage is for meats that are not organic but are not commercially raised either. Therefore, the animals are usually raised without growth hormones or antibiotics, but they can be fed and housed in any way. So, whereas natural is better than commercial, this is still not optimal.

◆ *Whole Grain*. Don't believe the label; look at the ingredient list. The word *whole* must appear before each grain in the list—not just before the first one or only one of them but in front of each grain. If it doesn't, then the food is not a whole grain.

- *Antibiotic-Free.* This is similar to the hormone-free category but applies to both poultry and red meats. Generally, the animals are given antibiotics so that the herds remain healthy even if several animals contract a disease. The thing that bothers me the most is that the antibiotic residue limits were raised several years ago by 600 percent. This means that the milk and the flesh can now contain many traces of the residue and still be considered safe. I would not eat food like that, and it's probably one of the biggest causes of antibiotic-resistant super-bugs. Always look for food that's labeled antibiotic-free.

- *DHA Enhanced.* This term generally applies to eggs. Several companies, aware of the health benefits of increased DHA (an omega-3 fatty acid) in the diet for cardiovascular disease protection and enhanced brain function, have started to give their chickens a feed that has been saturated with DHA. It sounds like a great idea on paper, but these chickens are fed grain, which isn't their natural food, and are also given a substance that's not naturally found in their diet. This is another great untested experiment on humans.

- *Farm Raised.* This applies to fish. This is not a healthy way to get fish and, in my opinion, should be avoided at all costs. Always buy wild fish. Fish farms are able to manipulate the color of the fish they sell. The fish are fed grains and antibiotics, and the conditions are often horrible. I have never been to a worse place than a fish farm. Yes, the fish are usually cheaper this way, but do what I do—buy only wild fish that is on sale that week.

- *Nitrates and Nitrites.* These are generally found in preserved meats such as hot dogs, cold cuts, bacon, and so on. Although these products taste really good, they are hazardous to our health. Therefore, I recommend that you buy only these types of meats that specifically say "nitrate-free" or "nitrite-free."

Healthy food may be just as illusory as good health, but if we start to demand better products and better labeling, we'll get it. It takes time, but let's keep at it. So, take a deep breath and go to the grocery store.

Choosing the Right Fats and Oils

This is an enormous topic and one I covered thoroughly in *The Hamptons Diet*. Here, I will attempt to quickly summarize the essentials of what you need to know in order to cook in the healthiest fashion.

✦ Don't use canola oil for anything. It is probably the unhealthiest oil on the planet. It was never tested for human consumption and is made from a genetically engineered seed. It is highly overprocessed and damaged. Any reports that you hear about its health benefits are for the unprocessed oil—something that is not in our food supply because it is too fragile and unfit for human consumption.

✦ Olive oil should only be used cold. It has a low smoke point so it cannot be heated without the formation of unhealthy free radicals. This is the most common misconception in American cooking. Chef Jeff Harter agrees with me on this point because he worked in Spain for many years and knows a good deal about olive oils. His kitchen used to have ten to fifteen different types of olive oils, all with different and varying flavors, depending on the region where the olives were grown and when they were harvested. He used these as finishing oils—something drizzled on the food or the plate *after* it was heated and cooked. A good olive oil must be in a dark glass bottle and must have the date it was produced stamped on the label. There is a lot of mislabeling in the olive oil world. Most of the inexpensive brands are blended with other, cheaper oils to make them more affordable. Italian olive oil is also a misnomer, as most of the cheaper oils simply pass through Italy or have someone Italian working at the company. The reason olive oil is healthy is its high levels of monounsaturated fat, polyphenols, and vitamin E. Macadamia nut oil is higher in each of those properties. I grew up using olive oil, and it pains me to say these things, but I have found you a safer and healthier alternative—macadamia nut oil.

✦ Choose a high smoke point oil. This is the temperature at which the oil starts to smoke. That signals that the fatty acids are starting to disintegrate, and the oil is starting to go bad or turn rancid. This should be avoided because at this point, free radical and trans-fatty acid formation begins to occur.

- Go for monounsaturated fats and oils. These are the omega-9 fatty acids. They have been proven to decrease the risk for developing cardiovascular disease by lowering cholesterol levels and raising healthy HDL levels. They help to maintain stable cell membranes and thus decrease risk for certain cancers—breast cancer in particular. Also, the omega-9 fatty acid, oleic acid, has been shown to increase basal metabolic rates by up to 10 percent in some studies. By substituting monounsaturated fat like macadamia nut oil for saturated and polyunsaturated fat—by switching cooking oils—you can lose more weight.

- Decrease the amounts of polyunsaturated cooking oils. These are the unhealthy and pro-inflammatory omega-6 fats. They are the most common cooking oils, such as corn, peanut, grapeseed, sesame, soybean, sunflower, and safflower oils. By consuming these types of oils, you increase your risk of developing heart disease, diabetes, and other inflammatory conditions such as arthritis and stroke.

- Keep saturated fats to a minimum. These fats have been shown to increase heart disease. They are found in coconut oil, other tropical oils, animal fat, margarine, butter, and ghee. Of these, ghee and butter are the most acceptable from a health perspective. Along with animal fat, they contain certain medium-chain triglycerides that have proven health benefits. So, although I say to keep them to a minimum, they need not be avoided altogether.

- Avoid hydrogenated oils and trans-fatty acids. These are by far the unhealthiest fats. They are found in packaged and processed foods. Also, when we eat out, these are the oils we are exposed to, primarily because restaurants tend to reheat oil all the time, and each time it is heated and cooled, trans-fatty acids form. As little as 3 grams per day of trans fats can significantly increase your risk for developing heart disease. The average doughnut contains 9 grams of trans fats. Think about that every time you are tempted to reach for a Krispy Kreme.

When choosing a cooking oil, select one with a high smoke point, low levels of pro-inflammatory omega-6 fatty acids, the ideal ratio of omega-6 to omega-3 fats, and the highest levels of monounsaturated omega-9 oleic acid. Since you will probably want to experience other cooking oils from time to time, or you may be allergic to nuts, I have included most of the common oils in the following chart so that you can use this as a guide. By the way, if you are using recipes from another cookbook, you can substitute macadamia nut oil for any other oil in the recipe and vice versa.

Key things to look for:

1. Highest smoke point, coupled with and not exclusive of

2. Low levels of polyunsaturated omega-6

3. High levels of monounsaturated omega-9

Cooking Oil Comparison				
Oil	Smoke Point	Monounsaturated Fat % (omega-9)	Polyunsaturated Fat % (omega-6)	Saturated Fat %
Corn*	320°F	27	59	13
Peanut	300°F	48	34	18
Sesame	300°F	40	45	15
Soybean*	300°F	24	56	15
Safflower	300°F	14	78	8
Olive*	300°F	72	12	15
Grapeseed	400°F	15	76	9
Canola*	350°F	54	24	12
Macadamia Nut*	410°F	84	2	12
Hazelnut	425°F	75	15	10
Coconut	450°F	8	1	91
Avocado	520°F	65	18	17
Sunflower	300°F	19	69	12
Almond	430°F	65	28	7
Walnut*	320°F	28	58	9

* Where percentages do not total 100 for an oil, the remaining quantities represent omega-3 fats.

Although you'll see recipes in this book that use various oils and fats, we did that simply for the sake of variety. After all, having a little of something, although not the healthiest ingredient, won't harm anyone. So, the bottom line is

1. Use macadamia nut oil for any type of heated cooking unless you are allergic to nuts. Since macadamia nuts are tree nuts, however, most people can tolerate this oil even though they may be allergic to peanuts. I must caution you, though, to try this only at your own risk. If you are allergic to peanuts and you try macadamia nut oil, have an epi-pen handy.

2. Use estate-bottled extra-virgin olive oil from a reputable source and expect to pay a lot of money for it—and use it only in cold dishes.

3. Use avocado oil if you are allergic to nuts or don't like macadamia nut oil for heating purposes. Hazelnut oil, if you are not nut-sensitive, is my second-favorite oil, and avocado takes third place.

4. Always avoid canola oil.

5. If, for whatever reason, you can't follow the previous suggestions for choosing a cooking oil, refer to the chart and just make the best selection you can, based on the criteria.

6. Use butter instead of margarine. It has good medium-chain triglycerides and doesn't contain harmful trans-fatty acids as margarine does (despite what you may read on the label, margarine still has them).

3

Hamptons Diet Breakfast Recipes

Cooking can be easy, but it's often frustrating and scary for most people. It doesn't have to be, and I encourage you to follow the simple steps outlined in this cookbook, so that you can make a quick, easy meal that is healthy and delicious any time you feel like it. Cooking doesn't have to be time consuming when you know a few simple steps.

Breakfast is the most important meal of the day. It gets our metabolism going. I find that if I eat a proper breakfast, I'm not as hungry the rest of the day. There is always time for breakfast, especially if you make it ahead of time and can eat it cold in the car, on the bus, or on the subway or can heat it up when you get to the office. Most of these recipes can be made ahead of time and kept in the refrigerator to eat for the rest of the week. The other thing I do is eat nontraditional breakfast foods, like turkey or salmon. Broaden your horizons—breakfast doesn't have to be bread and carbohydrate oriented. The carbohydrate recipes in this section all use slow-release carbohydrates and are low-glycemic-load meals. Please enjoy them as much as we did when we prepared them.

The first recipe in this book is a perfect illustration of cooking Hamptons style—that is, incorporating as many healthy foods into one meal as possible. The second principle is to offer a recipe where the main ingredient can be changed to any other similar ingredient, and you have a completely new dish. This way, you need to learn only a few recipes or tricks of the cooking trade, and people will think you have always known how to cook. For example, in this recipe, it's possible to change the berry topping and the flour used in the crepe. The recipe can give you at least twenty dishes simply by mixing and matching the berries and the flour, and each one will taste different—yet you've learned and mastered only one recipe.

Buckwheat Crepes with Mascarpone and Strawberries

SERVES 6–8.

The first time I made crepes, it wasn't pretty. The entire kitchen and part of the dining room were a mess, covered in flour. I spent about five hours trying to make the perfect crepe. I ran out to the store at least three times for more flour, and after using about fifteen pounds of flour, I had my first successful crepe. I was only fourteen at the time. It's going to be much easier for you to master this, I promise.

Jeff learned how to make these crepes from a friend when he was living in Spain. This is a wonderfully healthy, yet indulgent, breakfast. I have even served these at brunch, to many rave reviews. These crepes incorporate a nice whole grain and a fresh fruit. To make this dish perfect, simply serve it with some protein, like nitrate-free bacon or chicken-with-garlic sausages.

I love recipes where you can make things early and save them for a rainy or lazy day. These crepes can even be served cold as a great after-school snack.

2 tablespoons unsalted butter

1 cup heavy cream

¼ teaspoon salt

½ cup buckwheat or other whole-grain flour

1½ teaspoons macadamia nut oil

2 small eggs

¼ cup low-carbohydrate beer

1 cup mascarpone cheese

¼ teaspoon lo-han or other sugar substitute (see chapter 8 for a full description of recommended sugar alternatives)

1 cup fresh strawberries, sliced (use other berries if they are more seasonal or local)

Melt the butter in a small saucepan. Add the cream and salt, stir well, then remove from the heat.

Put the flour in a mixing bowl, make a well in the center, and pour in the oil and eggs. Mix the eggs and oil with a whisk, gradually bringing in flour from the sides until it begins to thicken. Add the cream mixture little by little until all of it has been added and the batter is smooth. Whisk in the beer. Pour the batter through a strainer into a bowl and refrigerate it for at least 2 hours before using. This batter can even be made a day ahead to save precious time in the morning.

Preheat a 10-inch nonstick skillet. Pour 1 tablespoon of macadamia nut oil in the skillet and wipe it off with a paper towel. Using a small ladle, pour about 1 fluid ounce of batter in one spot at the edge of the pan. Immediately tilt and swirl the pan, moving the batter around the pan down over the center, until the cooking surface is covered with the scant batter—remember, these are crepes, not pancakes. Make sure the pan isn't too hot. Your first crepes might not be perfect, but just keep trying. You'll get the hang of it.

Cook the crepe for about 1 minute per side. The first side is ready to be turned when you see the edges browning. Remove it from the skillet and repeat the process until the batter is finished. If you don't intend to use the crepes right away, cover them with plastic wrap and refrigerate.

Place the mascarpone in a large metal bowl and whip with a whisk for about 1 minute. Add the sugar substitute and whip for another 10 seconds.

To assemble, lay the crepe on a plate, spread 1 tablespoon of the mascarpone mixture down the middle of the crepe, and top with 2 tablespoons of strawberries. Fold both edges of the crepe over and serve. Top with more strawberries, if desired.

Good for B and C dieters.

Cantaloupe with Cottage Cheese and Seasonal Berries

SERVES 4.

Jeff's mother made this for his family when he was growing up. When these fruits are in season, this simple dish is sublime. This seasonal dish is great for lazy summer mornings.

1 ripe cantaloupe
1 cup cottage cheese
¼ cup blackberries
¼ cup blueberries
¼ cup boysenberries
¼ cup strawberries

Cut the cantaloupe in half and scoop out the seeds. Then quarter the melon.

In a large bowl, gently mix the cottage cheese and all the berries. Place each melon quarter on a separate plate and divide the berry mixture accordingly.

Good for A, B, and C dieters.

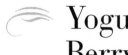

Yogurt and Mixed Berry Breakfast

SERVES 4.

This makes for a quick light snack or meal. Although yogurt is naturally high in sugar, if you get the natural, plain, and no-sugar versions, or even substitute kefir, it will make a healthy snack because the oat bran slows the absorption of sugar and makes this recipe low glycemic.

½ cup mixed berries (strawberries, raspberries, blueberries)
1 cup plain, nonsugar yogurt
½ cup oat bran

Place all the berries in a small bowl. Spoon the yogurt on top of the berries. Sprinkle the oat bran on top of the yogurt and serve immediately.

Good for B and C dieters.

Grandma's Granola

SERVES 8.

This recipe is adapted from one by Jeff's grandmother, Edna Harter. After his grandmother passed away, his stepmother gathered all of her recipes, photocopied them, classified them, and put them together to create a wonderful family cookbook.

2 cups rolled oats
½ cup chopped almonds
½ cup sesame seeds
½ cup sunflower seeds
¼ cup macadamia oil
¼ cup powdered lo-han

Preheat the oven to 325°F. Mix all the ingredients in a large bowl. Place the mixture on a cookie sheet and bake for 30 minutes, stirring the granola every 10 minutes. Allow the granola to cool or serve it warm and gooey.

Good for A, B, and C dieters.

The Basic Omelet

SERVES 2.

The first time I tried to roll an omelet, it was a complete disaster. I had a room filled with eggs and egg shells, grease stains everywhere, and eggs on every bit of the stove except in the pan. I remember my college roommate waking up after a long night of debauchery and not being able to remember whether the party had continued in our suite—it looked that bad. Of course, I told him the party had, so that he would help me clean up.

A general rule is two eggs per person when you're deciding how many eggs to use for a recipe. With omelets, though, you can usually subtract one egg from the amount you think you should use, as long as you keep all the other ingredients in the same proportions. For example, in this recipe Jeff is teaching us how to make an omelet for two using three eggs. If you wanted to make an omelet for four, use six eggs but double the rest of the ingredients that go into it. It may sound a little confusing, but you'll get it with practice. The number of eggs is really not that critical an issue.

Omelets are a perfect breakfast food, as well as a snack food that can be eaten either cold or reheated. They last up to one week in the refrigerator without spoiling. I generally make one huge omelet at the beginning of a week and then nosh from it the rest of the week. (For those of you who aren't from New York, nosh means "pick on" or "nibble.")

As you'll see in the next few pages, omelets are limitless in terms of what can go into them. They are a kitchen sink–type food. If you always keep eggs in the house, you can always have a good meal. Scramble some eggs and use whatever leftovers you have in the refrigerator. Throw them into the bowl, pour this into a skillet, add heat, and voila! A meal.

3 large eggs
Salt
2 tablespoons macadamia nut oil

Place a medium nonstick skillet over very low heat until a few drops of water boil on contact. Meanwhile, in a large bowl mix the eggs and a pinch of salt. Beat them enough to combine the yolks and whites, but don't overbeat. Jeff prefers to use a dinner fork and beats them about 40 to 50 times. When the eggs are ready, turn the heat to medium-high. Add the oil and tilt the pan to coat the sides with oil. When the oil is sizzling but not yet burning, add the eggs.

Wait about 10 seconds for a ring of puffy egg to form around the edges. Then, with a wooden spoon or heat-proof spatula, cut through and scramble the eggs for a few seconds. Let the eggs set again for about 10 seconds, scramble one more time, and then add your preferred ingredients.

Use your spatula to mass the cooked egg against the back slope of the pan. Then tip the pan a little more and give it a little yank, using your spatula to nudge the far edge of the mass to roll over. The idea is to repeat this process, creating a cocoonlike shape. Don't worry if it starts to break and leak; just keep rolling the omelet. The eggs will cook, and the wrinkles will look great. Repeat the rolling and tipping gestures until the omelet is cooked to your taste. Just remember that practice makes perfect.

Each of the following omelet recipes will serve two unless otherwise stated.

The All-American

Clearly, this omelet can be made with any kind of cheese you or your family likes. I think the cheese omelet is an American classic.

2 ounces cheddar cheese, grated

Add the cheese to the omelet at the appropriate time and cook as described in the Basic Omelet recipe.

Good for A, B, and C dieters.

The Roman

¼ cup sundried tomatoes, chopped
¼ cup mozzarella, grated
1 tablespoon fresh basil, chopped

Add the ingredients to the omelet, and cook as described in the Basic Omelet recipe.

Good for B and C dieters.

The Parisian

½ teaspoon fresh chives, chopped
½ teaspoon fresh parsley, chopped
½ teaspoon fresh thyme, chopped
½ teaspoon fresh scallion, chopped
2 ounces Gruyère cheese, grated

Mix the herbs and cheese together in a small bowl. Spoon these ingredients onto the omelet and cook as described in the Basic Omelet recipe.

Good for A, B, and C dieters.

The OC

2 slices bacon, uncured and nitrate-free
½ cup avocado
¼ cup chilled Brie cheese (rind removed), cut into ½-inch cubes

Cook the bacon in a medium skillet until crisp; drain on a paper towel. Crumble the bacon and set aside. For something really delicious but not particularly healthy, prepare the omelet as described previously but with some of the oil left over from cooking the bacon. (I would recommend you try this only if you are using organic bacon and then only once per lifetime!) Spoon the bacon, avocado, and cheese onto the omelet and continue cooking the omelet as described in the Basic Omelet recipe.

Good for A, B, and C dieters.

The Santa Fe

2 pieces bacon, uncured and nitrate-free
Pinch cayenne pepper
2 ounces Monterey Jack cheese, grated
½ tomato, chopped
¼ red bell pepper, chopped
¼ jalapeño pepper, chopped
¼ avocado, chopped

Cook the bacon in a medium skillet until crisp; drain on a paper towel. Crumble the bacon and set aside. Spoon the ingredients onto the omelet and continue cooking the omelet as described in the Basic Omelet recipe.

Good for A, B, and C dieters.

The Southampton

1 ounce smoked salmon
1 tablespoon salmon caviar
2 teaspoons fresh dill

Spoon these ingredients onto the omelet and cook as described in the Basic Omelet recipe.

Good for A, B, and C dieters.

The Welsh

2 slices bacon
1 tablespoon macadamia nut oil
½ apple, peeled, cored, and thinly sliced
2 tablespoons crumbled Stilton cheese

Cook the bacon in a medium skillet until crisp; drain on a paper towel. Crumble the bacon and set aside. Heat a medium skillet over medium heat with the oil. When the skillet is hot, add the apple and sauté until golden, about 3 to 4 minutes. Transfer the mixture to a bowl.

Spoon the bacon, apple, and cheese onto the omelet and cook the omelet as described in the Basic Omelet recipe.

Good for B and C dieters.

The Lyonnaise

2 tablespoons macadamia nut oil
1 to 1½ onions, very thinly sliced

Heat the oil in a large skillet and add the onions. Cook the onions for about 15 minutes until they release liquid. Turn the heat to high to evaporate the liquid. Stir constantly to prevent sticking and burning.

When all the liquid has evaporated, turn the heat to low and cook the onions another 15 minutes, stirring every 2 to 3 minutes. Spoon the onions onto the omelet and cook as described in the Basic Omelet recipe. A variation is adding cheese to this dish.

Good for A, B, and C dieters.

The Cape Codder

4 ounces shrimp, cooked, shelled, chopped
1 tablespoon crème fraîche
1 teaspoon fresh tarragon leaves, chopped

Mix the three ingredients in a bowl, then spoon this mixture onto the omelet and cook as described in the Basic Omelet recipe.

Good for A, B, and C dieters.

The Greek Omelet

SERVES 2.

This omelet is a little more complicated, so we dedicated a special recipe for it. It isn't too tricky but is certainly more involved than the previous ones. Try this one for yourself first.

2 tablespoons macadamia nut oil
½ cup button mushrooms, sliced
Salt
Black pepper, freshly ground
1 garlic clove, minced
¾ cup baby spinach
2 tablespoons feta cheese, crumbled
2–3 large eggs

Add 1 tablespoon of macadamia nut oil to a preheated medium nonstick skillet with low sloping sides. Wait for the oil to become hot, then add the mushrooms, salt, and black pepper. Cook over medium-low heat, stirring often, until the mushrooms turn a golden brown. Add the garlic and cook for 2 minutes more, stirring constantly. Add the cleaned baby spinach, stir once, and place the mixture in a bowl. Stir the crumbled feta cheese into the mushroom and spinach mixture. Set aside.

Put the eggs in a medium glass bowl. Add a grinding of pepper and a pinch of salt to taste. Gently beat with a fork until well blended.

Put the same skillet over medium heat for about 1 minute. Add the remaining tablespoon of macadamia nut oil to coat the pan. Pour the eggs into the pan, reduce the heat to low, and cook for about 10 seconds or until the bottom is set. Pick up the pan and swirl the egg mixture so that the eggs become evenly cooked. Turn the heat to low and continue cooking until the eggs are soft-set. All of this should take less than 2 minutes.

Place the filling in the middle of the omelet. Fold over the sides to cover the filling and place the omelet on a warm plate with the seam side down.

Optional: A dollop of sour cream and a sprinkle of chopped chives will put this omelet over the top.

Good for A, B, and C dieters.

Four-Onion Frittata with Sage and Asiago

Serves 4.

In Italy, Jeff used to make a grilled pizza with four onions and sage. The flavors that develop from using red onion, Spanish onion, leeks, and shallots are amazing. The Asiago cheese lends the frittata a slight tang, and the sage rounds out these flavors with its elegance.

2 tablespoons macadamia nut oil
1 medium Spanish onion, diced
1 small red onion, diced
1 large leek, white part only, diced
1 shallot, diced
Salt
White pepper, freshly ground
8 large eggs
2 tablespoons fresh sage, chopped
½ cup young Asiago cheese, grated

Preheat the oven to 375°F.

In a large nonstick (ovenproof) skillet with low, sloping sides, heat 1 tablespoon of the oil for about 2 minutes. Add the Spanish and red onions and sauté for 10 to 12 minutes, stirring occasionally. Add the leek and shallot. Season with salt and pepper and continue cooking over low heat for another 10 to 12 minutes or until the mixture is a light golden brown. Remove the mixture from the heat and place in a small bowl. Set aside.

In a large bowl, whisk the eggs until fully beaten; add more salt and pepper as needed. Add the onion mixture, sage, and cheese to the eggs and lightly mix with a fork.

Place the large nonstick (ovenproof) skillet over medium heat for 1 minute. Add the remaining tablespoon of oil and coat the skillet well, including the sides. Pour the mixture into the skillet, remove the skillet from the stove, and place it in the preheated oven. Bake for about 20 to 25 minutes or until the frittata's edges are brown and the center is set.

Good for A, B, and C dieters.

Cinnamon Cheesy Oatmeal

SERVES 4.

Although I hate to admit it, the five years I lived in Dallas did rub off on me. The cooking and the people were certainly something I was not used to. The people were very nice and the foods spicy and rich, without a lot of fuss. I have tried to adapt that way of thinking about cooking and meals. The first time I had cheese grits was at a diner in Dallas called Lucky's. It was a very popular place for Sunday brunch, and most times there were people lined up down the block for simple Southern cooking. This is a healthier version of that dish.

It's important to keep in mind that not every meal needs to be a feast. This simple recipe illustrates how easy it is to take something ordinary and give it a little more pizzazz—the Hamptons way. This is my version of grits with cheese served Southern Style.

Pinch salt
2½ cups water
1 cup steel-cut oats
⅓ cup lo-han, or stevia to taste (optional)
½ teaspoon cinnamon, ground
2 tablespoons Tabasco sauce
½ cup cheddar cheese, shredded

In a large saucepan, bring the salted water to a rolling boil. Add the oats and cook for about 20 minutes, stirring constantly. Transfer the oats from the saucepan to a large mixing bowl and add the remaining ingredients except the cheese. Mix thoroughly. Divide the mixture into four bowls and sprinkle equally with the grated cheese. You could serve the oatmeal this way immediately, or you could place the (heatproof) bowls under the broiler until the cheese gets crispy. Either way, this is an excellent way to start the day.

Good for B and C dieters.

Oat Bran Pancakes

SERVES 6 TO 8.

This recipe takes an old classic and turns it on its head, making it healthier in the process. Healthy eating no longer means having to eat really strange food that smells and tastes terrible. I have been practicing nutritional medicine for the last eleven years, and what a difference that time has meant! It's so easy to eat in a healthy way now, and the options are incredibly yummy.

There can be so many variations on this simple pancake recipe. You can puree berries to pour over the pancakes. You can dice apples and pears in the winter months to spoon over them. You just need to use your imagination and use whatever is fresh, local, and seasonal for the healthiest results.

Macadamia nut oil in a spray bottle
1 cup oat bran cereal, uncooked
½ cup whole wheat flour
¼ cup lo-han or 3 packets of stevia
1 teaspoon baking powder
½ teaspoon baking soda
Pinch salt
2 cups heavy cream
2 eggs

Heat a nonstick griddle that has been lightly oiled with macadamia nut oil over medium-high heat. Combine the oat bran, flour, sweetener, baking powder, baking soda, and salt in a large bowl. Set aside.

Beat the heavy cream and eggs in a small bowl with a wire whisk. Pour the egg mixture over the dry ingredients. Stir together until the ingredients are just blended and no large dry lumps appear.

Pour approximately ¼ cup of pancake batter onto a hot, lightly oiled griddle. Cook until the pancakes are puffed, browned, and slightly dry around the edges. Flip, then cook the other side until golden brown, about 2 minutes.

Good for A, B, and C dieters.

Scrambled Eggs with Ricotta Cheese and Basil

SERVES 4.

While in Italy, Jeff lived with two Italian guys in an apartment next to the restaurant he worked in. One of them, Gianluca, made these eggs every Saturday morning for the guys. The ricotta was made fresh daily right down the road. The flavor was delicate and soft. Gianluca told Jeff that the trick was not to overcook the eggs. They should be soft and creamy.

6 large eggs
1 cup whole-milk ricotta cheese, stirred to blend
Salt
Pepper, freshly ground
1 tablespoon macadamia oil
1 tablespoon fresh basil leaves, sliced finely
2 tomatoes, cored and thinly sliced (optional, in season)

Combine the eggs, ricotta, salt, and pepper in a bowl and beat until well blended. Add the oil to a preheated large nonstick skillet over a medium-low flame. Then add the egg mixture to the skillet and cook, stirring constantly, until the eggs are soft-set but still creamy, about 3 minutes. Do not allow the eggs to become curdlike. If they do, they are overcooked. Top with the basil and place tomato slices alongside the eggs, if you like.

Good for A, B, and C dieters.

Scrambled Eggs with Buckwheat Groats, Wild Mushrooms, and Mediterranean Herbs

SERVES 4.

Jeff grew up in Boulder, Colorado, in a vegetarian family and was exposed to a lot of unusual ingredients. Buckwheat groats (hulled buckwheat kernels) stood out because of their delicate nutty taste. They are as easy to cook as the pasta you are used to.

2 cups cooked buckwheat groats (room temperature)
3 tablespoons macadamia nut oil
½ cup onions, chopped
2 cups white button, cremini, shiitake, and portobello mushrooms, sliced
1 garlic clove, minced
Salt
Black pepper, freshly ground
¼ teaspoon cayenne pepper
1 tablespoon fresh thyme, minced
1 tablespoon fresh rosemary, minced
1 tablespoon fresh marjoram, minced
6 large eggs
1 tablespoon heavy cream
1 tablespoon chives, chopped

Pour 1 cup of buckwheat groats into 3 cups of boiling salted water. Cook, uncovered, stirring occasionally, for about 13 to 15 minutes or until tender. Rinse with cold water and let strain for 5 minutes. This will give you 3 cups of groats, but for this recipe you will need only 2 cups, so save 1 cup for another dish.

Place 2 tablespoons of macadamia nut oil in a large nonstick skillet over medium heat. When the oil is hot but not smoking, add the chopped onion and sauté for about 5 minutes or until translucent. Add the sliced mushrooms and sauté until lightly browned. Add the garlic, a sprinkle of salt, a dash of black pepper, the cayenne pepper, the herb mixture, and the buckwheat groats. Cook these ingredients for about 2 to 3 minutes, stirring occasionally. Reduce the heat to low.

In a medium bowl, whisk the eggs with the cream and a dash of salt and pepper. Using a spatula, push the buckwheat mixture to one side of the skillet. Place the remaining 1 tablespoon of macadamia nut oil in the center of the pan, and when it is heated, pour in the eggs. Cook until the eggs begin to set on the bottom, about 2 minutes. Cook, stirring gently, until they're soft-set but still creamy, about 2 minutes more. Carefully stir the eggs into the buckwheat mixture, trying not to break them up too much. When everything is heated through, about 2 minutes more, serve immediately and top with the chives.

Good for B and C dieters.

Huevos Revueltos à la Piperade

SERVES 4.

*Scrambled eggs are eaten throughout Spain for lunch or dinner but very seldom
for breakfast. Piperade is a tomato, red bell pepper, onion, and egg dish from the
Basque region of Spain. Jeff lived in this region for six months and worked at a
Michelin three-star restaurant there. This region is famous for its* pintxos *or*
tapas *(small plates), and he explored these wonderful* pintxo *bars on his days off.
One of his favorite places served huevos revueltos à la piperade on top of grilled
country bread. Here, we are not serving it on bread, although if you're a C dieter,
you certainly could if the bread was a true whole-grain bread.*

3 tablespoons macadamia nut oil
3 Spanish onions, cut in half and thinly sliced
2 green bell peppers, cut in half, seeded, and cut into ½-inch-wide strips
2 red bell peppers, cut in half, seeded, and cut into ½-inch-wide strips
¼ cup Canadian bacon, diced
1 garlic clove, minced
2 ripe tomatoes, blanched, peeled, cored, cut in half, seeded,
    and cut into ½-inch dice
1 teaspoon salt
White pepper, freshly ground
¼ teaspoon smoked Spanish paprika
8 large organic eggs

Heat the macadamia nut oil in a large nonstick skillet over medium-low heat.
Add the onions and cook, stirring, until tender, about 5 minutes. Add the bell
peppers and cook, stirring, until tender but not brown, about 10 minutes. Add
the Canadian bacon and garlic and cook 2 to 3 minutes. Add the tomatoes and
cook, stirring until the liquid has evaporated, 10 to 12 minutes. Add the salt,
pepper, and smoked Spanish paprika. Let simmer.

    Whisk the eggs in a bowl. Add the eggs to the skillet; reduce the heat to low
and cook, gently folding the eggs into the piperade with a spatula, until the
eggs are soft-set but still creamy, about 3 to 4 minutes. Serve immediately.

*If served without bread, good for A, B, and C dieters. If served with bread, good
only for C dieters.*

Cheese and Egg Casserole

SERVES 8 TO 10.

This recipe came to me through one of my Dallas patients. I lived in Dallas for five years. My patients there loved to cook and always had different twists on foods that I was used to making. Karen G. lost 24 pounds eating this way.

15 large eggs
2 cups heavy cream
1 teaspoon salt
1 teaspoon black pepper, coarsely ground
¾ teaspoon onion powder
2 tablespoons fresh chives, chopped
½ cup cheddar cheese, shredded

Whisk together the eggs and the rest of the ingredients, except the cheese, in a large bowl. Pour into a greased 8- × 10-inch baking dish. Stir in the cheese, then cover and chill the dish for 8 hours, stirring once. Preheat the oven to 350°F. Uncover the casserole and stir once more; then bake for 30 minutes or until it's set.

Good for A, B, and C dieters.

Alicante-Style Tortilla with Asparagus

SERVES 4.

Alicante is in the southern region of Spain on the Mediterranean coast. This Alicante-style tortilla is light, flat, and easy to make, unlike the dense potato-egg tortilla found throughout the rest of Spain. Here we are using pencil asparagus, but you can substitute any fresh vegetable.

24 pencil asparagus stalks
2 tablespoons macadamia nut oil
Salt
Black pepper, freshly ground
5 large eggs

Trim the asparagus stalks by cutting off the bottom third of the stalk. Cook in a saucepan in boiling salted water until just tender, 3 to 4 minutes. Remove to an ice bath to stop the cooking process. Drain well and place in a heated 12-inch nonstick skillet with 1 tablespoon of macadamia nut oil. Add a pinch of salt and pepper and sauté over medium heat for 2 minutes, stirring.

Meanwhile, in a small bowl, beat the eggs until well blended and season with salt and pepper. Shake the skillet so the asparagus spreads out evenly. Add the remaining oil to the skillet and pour the eggs over the asparagus. Place the skillet over medium-low heat, cover, and cook for about 2 minutes or until the top is just set. Slide the tortilla out onto a warm 14-inch plate. Cut into wedges and serve.

Good for A, B, and C dieters.

Eggs Benedict with Tom

This is Jeff's version of the all-American classic. Every cook needs to know to make this simple egg dish, and despite how easy it is to make, guests are always impressed.

4 thick slices large ripe tomato, in season
4 slices Canadian bacon
4 large eggs, poached (recipe follows)
1/4 cup prepared Hollandaise Sauce (recipe follows)

Preheat the oven to 400°F.

Place the tomato slices on a baking sheet and sprinkle with salt and pepper. Place a slice of Canadian bacon on top of each tomato and put the sheet in the oven for about 5 minutes until very hot.

Remove the tomato and the Canadian bacon from the oven and put them on plates. Place a poached egg on top of each slice of tomato and bacon. Then pour prepared Hollandaise Sauce on top of the egg and serve.

Poached Egg

This will teach you how to poach an egg, which can be used in many recipes in the book. It's the fancy chef's way of doing it, and believe me, it may take some practice. I probably messed up dozens of eggs trying to poach this way before I got the hang of it. I recommend trying this, as it does make a much better presentation than using an egg-poaching contraption. It will actually look like something from a restaurant.

Bring salted water to a raging boil in a small saucepan. Break one egg at a time into the water. You may need to spin the egg around in the boiling water to get the correct shape. The poaching process should take about 3 minutes, depending on how cooked through you prefer your yolks. For the Eggs Benedict dish, the yolks should be somewhat but not overly runny.

Good for A, B, and C dieters.

Hollandaise Sauce

MAKES 1½ CUPS.

½ pound butter
5 yolks
Juice of 3 lemons
Pinch cayenne pepper
Salt
White pepper, freshly ground

Melt the butter in a small saucepan. Place the yolks in a food processor or blender and blend on low speed until they double in volume. While the motor is still running, slowly add the hot melted butter. This cooks the yolks slightly. Then slowly add the lemon juice, cayenne, salt, and pepper. If the sauce is too thick, add a little water to thin it out. Correct the seasoning and keep the sauce warm until you're ready to use it.

Good for A, B, and C dieters.

Scrambled Eggs w
Bell Pepp<

This is a classic recipe, and you can use it with just about any vegetable combination you desire. The freshest, most seasonal vegetables you can find at the supermarket or the vegetable stand will be the best additions.

3 tablespoons macadamia nut oil
1 green bell pepper, cut into ¼-inch slices
1 orange bell pepper, cut into ¼-inch slices
1 yellow bell pepper, cut into ¼-inch slices
1 small clove garlic, minced
8 large eggs, beaten
Salt
Black pepper, freshly ground
2 tablespoons fresh Italian (flat-leaf) parsley, stems removed, chopped

Place the oil in a large nonstick skillet over medium-high heat. Add the bell peppers and sauté for about 3 to 4 minutes or until they have softened, stirring frequently. Add the garlic and cook for about 15 seconds. Add the beaten eggs to the skillet and scramble with a wooden spoon. Season with salt and pepper. Remove from the heat when they have reached your desired degree of doneness. Put the eggs on plates, then sprinkle with the parsley and serve hot.

Good for A, B, and C dieters.

Ham Roll-Ups with Poached Egg and Mornay Sauce

SERVES 4.

This dish is tasty in both the summer and the winter months. Asparagus is freshest in the late spring and the early summer, so that's usually when I serve this dish. The baked ham and the Swiss cheese give it a European flair. When I make it, I usually picture myself on the Champs-Elysées in Paris, as this is my version of a Croque Monsieur. As with most recipes in this book, you can vary it just by changing the cheese and the meat. I offer one suggestion—choose a sharp cheese so that it can hold up to the taste of the meat and the sauce.

8 slices baked ham
8 slices Swiss cheese
8 asparagus spears, cooked
Macadamia nut oil in a spray bottle
4 poached eggs (see recipe, page 57)
Mornay Sauce (recipe follows)

Preheat the oven to 350°F.

Place 2 ham slices overlapping slightly on a flat surface. Place 2 cheese slices over the ham. Top with 2 asparagus spears, then roll up. Repeat the process. Arrange the roll-ups in a lightly oiled baking dish. Place in the oven for 12 minutes. Place 2 roll-ups on each plate and top with a poached egg. Pour Mornay Sauce over the eggs and roll-ups.

Good for A, B, and C dieters.

Mornay Sauce
MAKES 1½ CUPS.

2 tablespoons butter
2 tablespoons whole wheat flour or other thickening agent*
1 cup heavy cream
½ cup Swiss cheese, shredded
Pinch nutmeg, freshly grated
Salt
Black pepper, freshly ground

Heat the butter in a saucepan over medium heat. Add the thickening agent and cook until bubbly. Lower the heat and stir in the cream. Cook until thickened. Stir in the cheese until the sauce is smooth. Stir in the nutmeg, salt, and pepper.

Good for A, B, and C dieters.

*Thickening agents can be many things. Most of the time, I use very dried cauliflower that I keep around the house for this occasion. I make the cauliflower according to the recipe in this book for mock potatoes on page 176, but don't add any of the condiments, butter, or cream. I simply boil the cauliflower, drain it thoroughly, and heat it in the oven several times until it's completely dry, and then place it in a sealed container. This can even be made in large batches and frozen in smaller ones so that you'll always have some on hand.

Guar gums or vegetable gums are a healthier way to thicken sauces without having to resort to flour. They take the place of the gluten in the flour, which is the thickening agent. You could also use unsweetened nut butters, but they will impart a specific taste, or simply add stock to the pan, deglaze it, and cook off most of the liquid on really high heat. Clearly, that is not meant for this recipe, but it's something to keep in mind for other sauces. What I'm really saying is, don't rely on your old standby techniques. Experiment with new ways to make your food choices and meals healthy.

Bacon and Egg "Muffins"

SERVES 6.

This is a great recipe for a brunch appetizer and also for people who lament not being able to have muffins in the morning. Muffins is often a marketing term for little slices of cake; these healthier muffins can be made ahead of time and eaten cold on the way out the door or heated when you arrive at the office. Kids also love them, and they make great snacks in-between practices, games, and other activities.

6 strips bacon
2 tablespoons macadamia nut oil
¼ cup Spanish onion, diced
6 eggs
2 tablespoons heavy cream
Salt
Black pepper, freshly ground
Macadamia nut oil in a spray bottle

Preheat the oven to 350°F.

Either place the bacon on a microwave-ready plate covered in paper towels to absorb the grease, and cook on high for about 4 minutes on each side—the bacon should be well done—or cook the bacon in a nonstick skillet until well done, about 20 minutes. Dice into small pieces, then set aside.

Heat 1 tablespoon of macadamia nut oil in a small skillet. Add the onion and sauté until golden, about 5 minutes. Set aside.

In a large mixing bowl combine the eggs, bacon, cheese, onion, heavy cream, salt, and pepper.

Spray a muffin pan with macadamia nut oil and spoon the mixture evenly into 6 compartments. Bake for 30 minutes, or until a toothpick comes out clean. Serve immediately or allow to cool in the pan for 10 minutes, then remove from the pan, place in a ziplock storage bag, and keep them in the refrigerator for later.

Good for A, B, and C dieters.

Eggs Florentine

This is Jeff's version of a classic European recipe he learned in Florence, which he thinks is the most romantic city he has ever visited. So get to work on this, and picture yourself and your lover strolling down the banks of the Arno River basking in the generous light of early morning and watching the mist recede into the hills, coating the olive trees with fresh dew.

2 tablespoons macadamia nut oil
2 tablespoons chopped onion
1 clove garlic, minced
½ pound cooked fresh spinach
Macadamia nut oil in a spray bottle
4 eggs
Mornay Sauce (see recipe, page 61)

Preheat the oven to 350°F.

Heat the oil in a skillet. Add the onion and garlic and cook until tender. Add the spinach and toss until mixed, about 1 minute. Do not overcook the spinach. Place the mixture in a baking dish that has been lightly sprayed with macadamia nut oil. Make four hollows in the spinach mixture and slip the eggs into the hollows. Cover with Mornay Sauce and bake for 10 minutes or until the eggs are set.

Good for A, B, and C dieters.

$$\approx 4 \approx$$

Hamptons Diet
Lunch Recipes

As a good rule for your health, you should eat three smaller meals each day and a couple of snacks. I personally find that difficult to live by because there just isn't enough time in the day to eat that much. Lunch for me is usually a salad from the deli downstairs near my office. On the weekends, however, or when I'm fortunate enough to be in the Hamptons during the week, lunch takes on more of an entertaining flair. This chapter consists of offerings for both leisurely lunchtimes and busy, during-the-week meals.

Roast Beef Roll-Ups

SERVES 4.

This is a classic quick lunch but with a slightly elegant flair. It incorporates vegetables into this time-honored dish. As presented this way, the roll-ups also make a colorful party appetizer good enough to serve to guests.

10 pieces of roast beef, from the deli (not prepackaged),
    freshly sliced thin
8-ounce package cream cheese
3 tablespoons horseradish
2 carrots, very thinly sliced
2 cucumbers, seeded and thinly sliced
1 red bell pepper, thinly sliced

Lay the roast beef slices out on a cutting board or plate. In a separate small bowl, mix the cream cheese and horseradish together. Spread the mixture on the beef. Place a few sticks of carrot, cucumber, and bell pepper on top of the cheese mixture. Roll up the beef slices and wrap in plastic, then refrigerate overnight. If these are for lunch, you don't need to wrap them overnight—simply throw them into your bag at this point. For a party, when you're ready to serve the roll-ups, unwrap the plastic wrap and slice them in half. Stand the roll-ups upright with the flat side on the bottom. Place on a tray for an elegant presentation.

Good for A, B, and C dieters.

Turkey Roll-Ups
Ham Roll-Ups

You may use any deli meat in this recipe. You can also change the cheese. I have used Swiss and provolone (my favorite because of the bite); even thinly sliced cheddar cheese works well here. You can include the vegetables or not, but any time you can incorporate more vegetables into your diet, the healthier you will be.

Good for A, B, and C dieters.

Turkey Wrap

Here is a fun sandwich idea that you can make ahead of time and take with you, send to school, or even keep in the refrigerator for when the kids come home from school and are starving. You can also take this with you for those in-between snacks when driving the kids from one practice to another.

2 tablespoons light cream cheese
Whole-grain tortilla, 8-inch diameter
2 ounces turkey slices
2 ounces Swiss cheese
1 iceberg lettuce leaf

Spread the cream cheese on half of the tortilla. Lay the turkey, cheese, and lettuce on top of the cream cheese. Fold in the sides of the tortilla, then roll into a cylinder shape. Wrap in plastic.

Before serving, slice the wraps at an angle in halves or even quarters, depending on how you wish to use this recipe, and remove the plastic wrap.

Good for A, B, and C dieters.

Spinach Parmesan Soup

SERVES 6.

I think soups are a wonderful dish for a light lunch. They are very filling and they can be reheated, and they're an easy way to eat all of those vegetables we need each day for optimal health. Soup can also easily be taken to the office in a thermos and reheated.

3 tablespoons macadamia nut oil
1 small Spanish onion, peeled and minced
3 cloves garlic, peeled and minced
1½ pounds spinach, stems removed, roughly chopped, rinsed,
    and left damp
Salt
Black pepper, freshly ground
1½ quarts chicken stock
½ cup Parmesan cheese, freshly grated

Heat the oil in a large heavy pot; add the onion and garlic and sauté until softened but not browned, about 5 minutes. Add the spinach to the pot and season with salt and pepper. Stir for a few minutes until the spinach wilts but is still bright green. Add the stock, bring to a boil, remove from heat, and set aside until you're ready to serve. To finish, heat up a portion and add grated Parmesan to taste. Finish the soup with a drizzle of macadamia nut oil on top, or better yet, serve it with a cruet of macadamia nut oil so that your guests can use as much as they want.

Good for A, B, and C dieters.

Chicken Salad with Macadamia Nuts and Avocado

SERVES 4.

This is probably the most monounsaturated-rich dish in the book. It has incredibly healthy ingredients and makes a perfect lunch. It can be made ahead of time so that it can be taken to work or school.

4 6-ounce chicken breasts, boneless, skinless, cut into thin paillards
Salt and pepper, to taste
4 eggs, beaten
2 ounces heavy cream
Salt
Black pepper, freshly ground
4 ounces macadamia nuts, pulverized
1 cup macadamia nut oil
4 cups of mesclun greens mix
1 red bell pepper, julienned
1 yellow bell pepper, julienned
Chicken Salad Dressing (recipe follows)
2 medium avocados

Lightly season each chicken breast with salt and pepper. In a separate bowl, beat the eggs, cream, salt, and pepper well. Dip the chicken into the beaten eggs, then into the macadamia nuts. Repeat until all the breasts are coated. Pour the oil into a large skillet and heat until it's just below burning. Pan fry the chicken over medium-high heat for 3 to 4 minutes on each side until cooked through. Remove from the heat and set aside.

Place the salad greens and bell peppers in a separate wooden bowl and toss them with the dressing. Divide the salad into individual plates, pit and cut in half each avocado, and place one half decoratively on the side of each plate. Place one chicken breast on top of each salad and serve. The chicken can be served hot, warm, room temperature, or even cold. This salad is a true classic.

Good for A, B, and C dieters.

Chicken Salad Dressing

MAKES 1½ CUPS.

1 cup macadamia nut oil
¼ cup white balsamic vinegar (lemon juice would do, too)
1 tablespoon Pommery mustard
¼ cup scallions, white part only, chopped
Salt
Black pepper freshly ground

Combine all the ingredients in a stainless steel bowl and mix well.

The Ultimate Chicken Salad Sandwich

SERVES 1.

A famous actor once said to me that his favorite food was sandwiches. I would bet that many of you feel the same way but question why and how a sandwich fits in a cookbook made to accompany the Hamptons Diet. First, this is not a low-carbohydrate diet, but simply a controlled and healthy carbohydrate diet. The trick is to find a whole-grain bread that the family likes or buy more than one brand of bread if that's what it takes to keep everyone happy and healthy.

Who doesn't like a good chicken salad sandwich? Jeff has devised one basic recipe with multiple variations. Feel free to add whatever you or your child likes to the basic recipe.

1½ cups cooked chicken, minced
¼ cup maconnaise (see recipe, page 73)
Salt
Black pepper, freshly ground
Pinch of cayenne pepper
2 slices whole wheat bread or 1 whole wheat tortilla

In a small mixing bowl, combine all the ingredients until well blended. Spread the salad on whole wheat bread or a whole wheat tortilla.

The Palm Beach

Add ¼ cup of minced celery and 1 tablespoon of minced onion to the basic recipe.

The Sleepy Hollow

Add ¼ cup of minced celery, ¼ cup of minced apples, and 2 tablespoons of chopped walnuts to the basic recipe.

The Montrealer

Add ½ cup of minced ham and 1 teaspoon of Dijon mustard to the basic recipe.

The Pig Pen

Add ½ cup of crisp crumbled bacon to the basic recipe.

The Nogales

Add ½ cup each of chopped red and green bell peppers, 1 tablespoon of chopped red onion, and 1 teaspoon of paprika to the basic recipe.

The Kerala

Add ½ cup of chopped, toasted almonds and 1 teaspoon of curry powder to the basic recipe.

The Saigon Special

Add ½ cup of chopped water chestnuts, 1 teaspoon of minced ginger, and 1 tablespoon of soy sauce to the basic recipe.

The Sonoran

Add 1 tablespoon of seeded and minced jalapeño, 1 teaspoon of chili powder, and 1 teaspoon of minced cilantro to the basic recipe.

The Mediterranean

Add 1 chopped tomato and 1 tablespoon of chopped fresh basil to the basic recipe.

The Santa Barbara

Add 1 chopped avocado and ½ cup of arugula to the basic recipe.

Each of the Ultimate Chicken Salad variations is suitable for B or C dieters. You can use these ideas as the basis for any sandwich. You can begin with tuna or salmon from a can, or you can start with any other meat.

Maconnais

This wonderful recipe can be used as a sauce or accompaniment for just about any dish. It is a mayonnaise made with macadamia nut oil and very easy to make. Note that you must use a food processor or the recipe will not work correctly. If you use a blender, then you must use whole eggs, not just yolks. You can make many variations on this mayonnaise just by adding different herbs, spices, or even hot sauces.

3 egg yolks
Juice of ½ lemon
1⅓ cups macadamia nut oil

Place the yolks and lemon juice in the bowl of a food processor. Turn on the machine and slowly drizzle in the oil until the mixture is thick and emulsified. Season the mayonnaise with salt and pepper. To make different flavors, add your favorite herbs: tarragon, chive, basil, and so on.

Good for A, B, and C dieters.

Chicken Salad, Boulder Style

SERVES 6.

Jeff tells us that his dad made the best chicken salad in the world when he was a kid. He used the barbecued chicken from the night before, or, after Thanksgiving, he used turkey in this flavorful salad. Now that I've tasted this, I would have to agree with him. This is an outstanding preparation and not that difficult to make. I love this any time of the year, but since it's a simple preparation and doesn't require use of the oven, I like to make this recipe for the beach, at a picnic, or just poolside with friends.

Jeff uses his father's mayonnaise recipe, but you can also use the maconnaise recipe (see page 73) to change things up a bit. With this one recipe, you can make many variations—all delicious.

6 cups chicken, skinless, boneless, cooked and cut into small pieces
Salt
White pepper, freshly ground
2 tablespoons extra-virgin olive oil
3 tablespoons fresh lemon juice
½ cup fresh parsley, chopped
1 teaspoon fresh tarragon, chopped
2 ribs celery, chopped
½ cup scallions, white part only, chopped
¾ cup walnuts, chopped
1 cup Jeff's Homemade Mayonnaise (recipe follows)
1 head romaine lettuce, washed and dried
2 hard-boiled eggs, sliced

In a big mixing bowl, toss the chicken with the salt, pepper, oil, lemon juice, and herbs. Add the celery, scallions, and walnuts and toss some more. Cover and refrigerate the chicken salad for at least 15 minutes.

When you're ready to use the salad, drain any liquid, correct the seasoning, and add enough mayonnaise to bind the ingredients. Divide the romaine lettuce equally on six plates and top with chicken salad and a slice of egg.

Good for A, B, and C dieters.

Jeff's Homemade Mayonnaise
MAKES 1½ CUPS.

This dressing livens up any salad or sandwich. It's so easy to make and so much better when you make it at home. Jeff has informed me that the name mayonnaise *comes from Mahon, the principal city of the Balearic island of Minorca off the southeastern coast of Spain. I will now drop that information into as many conversations as I can.*

The beauty of homemade mayonnaise, as with maconnaise, is that you can add so many different spices to it to create any flavor you want. Think of it as the tabula rasa of the cooking world. It is textural and will take on any flavor you add. With so many spices available, the flavor combinations are endless and will change the recipe each time.

1 whole egg
1 egg yolk
¼ teaspoon mustard
Salt
2 tablespoons lemon juice
½ cup extra-virgin olive oil
½ cup macadamia nut oil

Place the egg, yolk, mustard, salt, and lemon juice in a food processor or blender. Blend for a few seconds. With the motor running, very slowly pour in the olive oil and then the macadamia nut oil until the mixture thickens. I've found that if you use a food processor, you can get away with just the one extra yolk. If you use a blender, you may need two whole eggs. It has something to do with how quickly the blades turn and how well they can emulsify.

Good for A, B, and C dieters.

Tropical Key Lime
Chicken Salad

SERVES 4.

It always amazes me that there are probably as many variations on cooking the same ingredients as there are people on the planet—probably even more. I love it when people send me recipes that I never would have thought of myself. This is one example.

2 chicken breasts, boneless, skinless
½ teaspoon salt
3 tablespoons macadamia nut oil
½ cup unsweetened Key Lime Juice (fresh or bottled)
8 cups salad greens, romaine or mixed
3 plum tomatoes, diced
1 avocado, diced
½ cup ranch dressing, sugar-free
½ cup macadamia nuts, chopped

Pound the chicken breasts until thin. Combine the salt, 2 tablespoons of macadamia nut oil, and the lime juice in a bowl and marinate the chicken breasts in this mixture for 1 to 2 hours.

Heat 1 tablespoon of oil in a skillet over medium heat. Add the chicken breasts and cook for 4 minutes on each side, until browned and cooked through. (The lime juice will caramelize a little bit.)

Put 2 cups of greens in each of 4 salad bowls. Divide the tomato and avocado among them. Chop the chicken breasts and place on top of the salads. Drizzle ranch dressing over each salad, and finish with a sprinkling of chopped macadamia nuts. The combination of crisp veggies, creamy avocado, tart and savory chicken, and crunchy nuts is out of this world!

Good for A, B, and C dieters.

Chinese Chicken Salad with Tamari/Macadamia Dressing

SERVES 4–6.

1 broiler-fryer (about 3 pounds, free range, if possible) or
    4 large chicken breast halves
4 cups lower-sodium chicken broth or water
Handful celery tops
1 teaspoon sea salt
6 peppercorns
1½ cups Tamari/Macadamia Dressing (recipe follows)
1 bunch fresh broccoli (organic, if possible), about 4 cups
6 cups organic baby greens
1 cup celery, chopped
4 green onions, sliced on a slant
5 large radishes, thinly sliced
½ red bell pepper, sliced into thin strips
½ cup macadamia nuts, toasted, unsalted

Simmer the chicken with the broth or water, celery tops, salt, and peppercorns in a large stock pot for approximately 1 hour or until the juices run clear when the meat is pierced. Drain and cool the chicken enough to handle it. Remove the skin and pull the meat from the bones. Cut the meat into bite-size pieces and put into a shallow baking pan.

Pour ¼ cup of Tamari/Macadamia Dressing over the chicken. Cover and chill for at least 1 hour (24 hours is best).

Trim the broccoli into neat florets and steam until just tender and still very bright green. Remove from the heat and place in an ice bath to stop the cooking process. (You could use them raw.) Let the water vapor come off the broccoli, and then put the florets into a shallow pan. Pour ⅓ cup of Tamari/Macadamia Dressing over the broccoli florets. Cover and marinate but only for 1 to 2 hours. They get squishy if left overnight.

When ready to serve the dish, pile the salad greens, celery, green onions, radishes (save a few radish slices for garnish), and red pepper into a large shallow salad bowl. Pour the remaining Tamari/Macadamia Dressing over the salad and toss lightly to mix.

On individual chilled salad plates, divide the greens equally. Arrange the broccoli with the stems toward the center in a ring on top. Fill the ring with the marinated chicken. Top the chicken with toasted macadamia nuts.

Tamari/Macadamia Dressing

MAKES 1½ CUPS.

½ cup tamari sauce
½ cup macadamia nut oil
⅓ cup rice wine vinegar
1 teaspoon ginger, freshly grated
½ teaspoon garlic powder

Combine all of the ingredients in a jar with a tight-fitting lid. Shake well to mix. As you make this dressing, you can vary the amount of oil, vinegar, and tamari. You could even add a touch of stevia for a sweeter flavor.

Good for A, B, and C dieters.

Shellfish Cocktail

SERVES 12.

This dish comes from Andalucia in the southern part of Spain, where the seafood is incredibly fresh. What's great about this dish is that you can use whatever seafood you like or whatever was caught fresh that day.

8 ounces shrimp
8 ounces crabmeat
8 ounces lobster meat (1½-pound lobster)
20 mussels
8 ounces bay scallops
2 red onions, diced
2 green bell peppers, diced
2 red bell peppers, diced
¼ cup aged sherry vinegar
1 tablespoon salt
1 teaspoon white pepper, freshly ground
½ cup macadamia nut oil

You can buy precooked shrimp, crab, and lobster meat, but I wouldn't recommend it. If you are using fresh shellfish, bring salted water to a boil in a large pot. Drop in the shrimp and cook until pink, about 2 to 3 minutes. Take out the shrimp and place under cold running water until chilled. Place the lobster in the same boiling water and cook for 7 minutes. Remove from the boiling water and place under cold running water until chilled. Now put the mussels and bay scallops in the same water and boil for 2 to 3 minutes until all the mussels have opened. Unopened mussels should be discarded. Strain the mussels and bay scallops and run under cold water until chilled. Crabmeat is so much easier to buy precooked, so for this dish, I'll let it slide.

In a large glass bowl, add the sherry vinegar, salt, and pepper, and mix until the salt is dissolved. Slowly pour the macadamia nut oil into the vinegar while whisking vigorously. Place all the shellfish and vegetables in the bowl with the vinegar and oil. Toss well. Refrigerate the cocktail for about 1 hour until well chilled.

Serve on top of lettuce or chilled endive, if desired.

Good for A, B, and C dieters.

Main Beach Fish Chowder

SERVES 8.

Renee from East Hampton sent me this recipe. She always loved a good fish chowder but thought the typical variations could be enhanced. Here is her version. There are a lot of ingredients, but it's a very simple preparation. All the ingredients were local.

2 tablespoons macadamia nut oil
2 celery stalks, diced
2 garlic cloves, minced
1 bay leaf
4 cups chicken stock
2 cups heavy cream
6 ounces flounder or haddock fillets
4 large scallops
12 shrimp, medium sized
2 tablespoons fresh parsley, chopped
1 teaspoon tarragon, chopped
2 tablespoons chives, chopped
4 ounces bacon, diced and sautéed until crisp
Salt
Black pepper, freshly ground

In a medium saucepan over low heat, heat the oil and add the celery, garlic, and bay leaf. Cover and cook for about 5 minutes. Add the chicken stock and heavy cream and bring to a simmer. Add the flounder or haddock and cook gently until the fish is tender, about 3 minutes. Add the scallops and shrimp, and simmer until they are opaque, about 2 minutes. Discard the bay leaf and add the chopped herbs and bacon. Add salt and pepper to taste. Serve the chowder hot in small mugs.

Good for A, B, and C dieters.

Tangy Cucumber (or Zucchini) and Tuna Wrap

SERVES 4.

There is nothing more satisfying than a good tuna fish sandwich, especially one with a great little twist. These sandwiches are perfect to send to the beach in a little cooler or serve to the kids poolside. They're light and refreshing and won't weigh you down before that afternoon surf. They can be made ahead of time and taken out of the refrigerator when you're ready to serve them. You can also change the lettuce leaf or the vegetable inside the wrap to make this recipe your own and to keep the kids and the guests guessing.

2 cans (6 oz. each) chunk light tuna in water, drained
1 cucumber, sliced very thin, or ½ cup fresh zucchini, chopped
¼ cup red onion, chopped and rinsed under cold water
2 tablespoons fresh parsley, chopped
1 tablespoon capers, drained and rinsed
1 tablespoon Dijon mustard
3 tablespoons mayonnaise or maconnaise (see recipe, page 73)
Salt
White pepper, freshly ground
4 leaves of your favorite lettuce
4 whole-grain tortillas

In a large bowl, combine the first nine ingredients and mix well. Lay out a tortilla, place a lettuce leaf on it, and then add a quarter of the tuna mixture. Spread the mixture evenly to about a quarter inch from the edges. Fold in the top and bottom of the tortilla about an inch, and roll up tight. Wrap the tortilla in plastic wrap and refrigerate until you're ready to eat it.

Good for B and C dieters.

Southampton Crab Cakes

SERVES 4 FOR DINNER. SERVES 16 FOR APPETIZERS.

Every Christmas Day, I go to my friend Fran's home for brunch. Fran is one of the best cooks I have ever known and the author of a best-selling cookbook. She can make things taste really fattening and delicious, and you'll still lose weight eating her food. She has allowed me to use several of her newest recipes in this book.

½ pound lump crabmeat*
½ cup pecans, ground in food processor (¾ cup for appetizer)
Salt
1 tablespoon fresh chives, minced
2 tablespoons sour cream
2 tablespoons macadamia nut oil (for appetizers you will need 3)
6 large shallots, sliced
16 leaves flat-leaf parsley

Place the crabmeat in a mixing bowl. Add ¼ cup of the pecans and the salt, chives, and sour cream. Blend well. Heat the oil in a skillet. Add the shallots. Sauté over medium heat for about 3 minutes.

For appetizers, form the crabmeat mixture into balls the size of walnuts. Roll the balls in the remaining pecans. Flatten the balls into the shape of small burgers and place in the oil. (For a main dish, make four burger-shaped crab cakes and cook for 5 minutes on each side.) When all the crab cakes have been placed in the oil, cover the pan and allow the cakes to cook through for 3 minutes.

Remove the cover, gently turn over each crab cake (you don't want them to fall apart) and brown on the other side for 1 minute. Carefully remove the cakes from the pan and spoon the pan juices over them. Allow to sit for 5 minutes before serving. Garnish the appetizers with a piece of flat-leaf parsley.

Good for A, B, and C dieters.

*Crab substitute does not have the flaky texture or the flavor of real lump crabmeat. If for some reason you cannot use real crabmeat, use white albacore tuna that has been packed in water.

Simmered Shrimp with Shiitake Mushrooms and Scallions

SERVES 6.

This dish is very easy to make and shrimp make a perfect summer weekend lunch—sophisticated yet simple.

3 tablespoons macadamia nut oil
2 cloves garlic, thinly sliced
4 large shiitake mushroom caps, thinly sliced
½ cup scallions, white part only, diced
¼ cup white wine
1 cup chicken broth
1 teaspoon lemon juice
3 tablespoons butter
2 pounds large shrimp, peeled, deveined, and butterflied
2 tablespoons parsley, chopped
2 tablespoons basil, chopped
Salt
Black pepper, freshly ground

Put the oil in a large sauté pan over medium-high heat. Sauté the garlic for 1 minute, add the shiitake mushrooms and sauté for 1 minute, then add the scallions and sauté for 1 minute. Turn the heat to high and add the white wine. Cook everything for an additional minute, then add the chicken stock. Add the lemon juice and butter until the mixture is emulsified. Turn the heat down to low, to a gentle simmer; immerse the shrimp in the cooking medium and cook them 3 minutes on each side. Finish the dish with the parsley and basil and add salt and pepper to taste.

Good for A, B, and C dieters.

Poached Salmon with
Fennel Relish

SERVES 4.

Make sure you buy wild salmon. Because salmon is a seasonal fish, by the end of the winter all the fresh wild stock is gone. Only eat salmon at that time of the year if you can really trust your fishmonger.

You can do so many things with salmon. Poaching salmon is a great way to serve it on a hot summer afternoon. It goes well with a nice spinach salad.

3 cups water
1 cup dry white wine
1 teaspoon fennel seeds, coarsely chopped
1 bay leaf
1 tablespoon whole white peppercorns
1 lemon, cut into 4 sections
2 4-ounce, 1-inch-thick salmon fillets, without the skin
1 cup cucumber, peeled, seeded, chopped
½ cup fennel, chopped
½ cup green onion, chopped
½ cup radish, chopped
2 tablespoons sour cream
1 tablespoon Dijon mustard
Salt
White pepper, freshly ground

Bring the first six ingredients to a simmer in a heavy saucepan over low heat. Let steep for 15 minutes and then strain into a bowl. Return the liquid to the same pan and bring to a boil. Turn off the heat. Add the salmon and cook for 5 minutes per side. Using a slotted spatula, transfer the salmon to a baking sheet. Cover and refrigerate. This can be made a day ahead.

Combine the remaining ingredients in a small bowl. Season with salt and pepper to taste. Cover and refrigerate for at least 2 hours. When you're ready to serve the dish, place the salmon on plates. Spoon the relish over the salmon and serve.

Good for A, B, and C dieters.

Grilled Fish Chunks

This is another great summer barbecue recipe sent by a fan from Alabama. Helen K. had an awful time trying to lose weight until she discovered the Hamptons Diet and couldn't believe how easy it was to be healthy and lose weight all at the same time.

2 pounds thick fish, cut into large chunks (tuna, swordfish,
    mahi-mahi, or similar)
½ cup macadamia nut oil
2 cloves garlic, minced
Salt
Black pepper, freshly ground
1 tablespoon fresh oregano
Juice of 1 lemon
Fresh parsley leaves, chopped

This meal can be cooked in the broiler or on a grill. Heat the grill so that the fire is quite hot. The rack should be about 3 inches away from the heat. Thread the fish onto premoistened wooden skewers and brush the fish with some of the oil.

In a bowl, combine the garlic with the remaining oil, salt, pepper, and oregano and mix thoroughly. The ingredients can also be run through a food processor or blender to get a thin consistency. Add the lemon juice and set the mixture aside.

Grill the fish on each side for about 2 minutes. Brush the fish with the sauce and remove from the heat. Garnish with the parsley.

Good for A, B, and C dieters.

I know many of you will be surprised to find this heading in a healthy lower carbohydrate cookbook, but these are a secret and amazingly delicious set of dishes from Chef Jeff.

Beet and Goat Cheese Ravioli

SERVES 4.

I tend to serve these creative ravioli at lunchtime or as a first course during dinner. That way, four ravioli per person do the trick, you get people to enjoy vegetables in fun and creative ways, and it cuts down on the number of calories you are serving.

The beet replaces the pasta in these ravioli. This is a technique Jeff learned while in Spain working with Ferran Adria, considered to be the most creative chef in the world. For these creations, you will need a mandolin, Japanese or French, which I described in the kitchen equipment section of the book.

Once you have learned the technique, you can be creative and invent your own ravioli. A perfect example of cooking Hamptons style: one basic recipe and many delicious and healthy dishes.

1 large red beet
1 tablespoon macadamia nut oil
Salt
Black pepper, freshly ground
½ cup water
1 cup soft goat cheese
1 cup frisée salad, rinsed and dried
1 tablespoon fresh chives, chopped
¼ cup balsamic vinaigrette (see also the various vinaigrette
    recipes in chapter 6)

Preheat the oven to 375°F.

Rub the beet with oil and place in a deep baking dish. Season with salt and pepper, add the water, and cover the dish with foil. Place the dish in the oven for about 90 minutes or until a toothpick pierces the beet easily. Remove from the oven and let sit for about 5 minutes. Then, with a clean dish towel, take off the outer skin and place the beet in the refrigerator for about 1 hour.

When you're ready to make the ravioli, prepare the mandolin as per the instructions and slice the beet as thinly as possible until you are about a quarter of the way into the beet and you have a good diameter of the sliced beet to make the ravioli. The slices of beet must be wide enough to hold a filling, so you may have to discard the early part of the beet because the slices will be too narrow to use.

On a cookie sheet or baking tray (you may need more than one), lay out 32 beet slices side by side, with the matching sized slices next to each other. Place 1 tablespoon of cheese in the middle of each of 16 slices, then top with the matching slice. Place the ravioli in the oven for 2 to 3 minutes until warm but not hot.

Meanwhile, mix the frisée, chives, and half the vinaigrette in a large bowl.

Place ¼ cup of the frisée mixture in the middle of each plate. Then place four ravioli around the salad and pour the remaining vinaigrette over the ravioli.

Good for A, B, and C dieters.

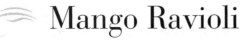

Mango Ravioli

SERVES 4.

Jeff recommends that you serve these ravioli as the appetizer course to his three main fish recipes, described in the dinner chapter.

2 ripe mangos
1 tablespoon macadamia nut oil
1 leek, white part only, finely chopped
½ jalapeño, seeded and finely chopped
½ pound peeled shrimp, finely chopped
Juice and zest of 1 lime
¼ cup cilantro, chopped
Salt
White pepper, freshly ground

Peel the mangos. Set up your mandolin—please read the instructions carefully—and slice the mangos as thinly as possible.

Place a medium skillet over medium heat and add the oil. Once the oil is hot, add the leeks and jalapeño and cook for about 5 minutes, stirring frequently and making sure not to brown the leeks. Then add the shrimp and cook for another 5 minutes or so. Add the lime juice and zest, cilantro, and salt and pepper. Take the shrimp off the heat, put them in a bowl, and refrigerate before you make the ravioli. This could take several hours, so the ravioli filling can be made ahead of time and stored in the refrigerator, even overnight.

When you're ready to serve the dish, place 1 tablespoon of filling on one-half of a mango slice, then fold the other half over. Repeat the process until all the filling is used up. Serve the ravioli cold.

Good for A, B, and C dieters.

Pineapple Ravioli

Jeff serves this as a midcourse intermezzo—a fancy term for a palate-cleansing snack between courses (hey, this is the tony Hamptons)—but I have served these ravioli as a dessert, as well as for breakfast or lunch. They are light and perfect in the middle of a day in early summer when the mint is at its freshest in the garden.

1 small pineapple
1½ teaspoons fresh mint, chopped
1 cup plain unsweetened yogurt

Peel the pineapple and set up your mandolin according to the instructions. Slice the pineapple as thinly as you can. In a separate bowl, stir the chopped mint into the yogurt. Put a tablespoon of the mixture in the middle of each pineapple slice and fold in the corners to create a ravioli. The ravioli can be refrigerated until you're ready to serve them.

Good for C dieters.

Vegetable Frittata with Manchego Cheese

SERVES 4.

Once you learn the technique of making a frittata, the only thing holding you back is your imagination, the seasonality of the vegetables, and your own taste buds.

1 tablespoon macadamia nut oil
1 small red onion, chopped
1 small red bell pepper, chopped
1 small zucchini, chopped
1 cup (packed) spinach leaves
6 eggs
Salt
Black pepper, freshly ground
1 ounce Manchego cheese, grated

Preheat the oven to 400°F.

Heat the oil in a 10-inch nonstick ovenproof skillet over medium heat. Add the onions and cook for 5 minutes or until translucent. Add the bell pepper and cook for another 5 minutes. Add the zucchini and cook the vegetables for another 5 minutes. Add the spinach and cook until it's wilted.

Beat the eggs in a large bowl with salt and pepper. Add the vegetables to the eggs, and mix well. Pour the mixture back into the hot skillet and set over medium-low heat. Cook until the eggs are set on the bottom of the skillet, about 5 minutes. Sprinkle the frittata with cheese and place the skillet in the oven. Bake for about 5 to 10 minutes or until the eggs are cooked all the way through. Serve the frittata warm with a mixed salad.

Good for A, B, and C dieters.

Blue Cheese Terrine

SERVES 12.

Kevin S. sent this recipe to me from the Hamptons. It's an elegant little party starter with visual appeal, and it contains ingredients that he could get locally. Kevin has now dropped 74 pounds and looks terrific. Kevin uses a tomato basil vinaigrette, but you can substitute whatever salad dressing you prefer.

2 red bell peppers, cut in half
2 yellow bell peppers, cut in half
6 ounces blue cheese, crumbled
2 8-ounce packages cream cheese, softened
Tomato Basil Vinaigrette (recipe follows)
Mixed salad greens

Preheat the oven to broil. On an aluminum foil–lined baking sheet, place the red and yellow bell peppers cut sides down and broil 5 inches from the heat for about 8 minutes until the peppers look blistered. Place the peppers in a ziplock bag, seal it, and let sit for about 10 minutes to loosen the skins. Peel the skins off the peppers and pat the peppers dry.

Beat the cheeses with an electric mixer on medium until the mixture is smooth. Spread half of the cheese mixture in a plastic wrap–lined 8- × 4-inch loaf pan. Top with 4 pepper halves. Spread the remaining cheese mixture over the peppers and top with the remaining pepper halves. Chill for 8 hours.

Unmold onto a serving dish and drizzle your favorite dressing over it. Carve and serve the slices over mixed greens.

Tomato Basil Vinaigrette

MAKES 2 CUPS.

¼ cup white wine vinegar
1 tablespoon Dijon mustard
1 teaspoon salt
½ teaspoon black pepper, freshly ground
1 teaspoon lime juice
½ cup macadamia nut oil
¼ cup fresh basil, chopped

Whisk together the first five ingredients in a small bowl. Gradually mix in the oil, then add the fresh basil.

Good for A, B, and C dieters.

Moroccan Beef Kabobs

SERVES 6.

This is a low-fat and low-carbohydrate meal. It makes a great lunch when you're sitting by the pool or a great appetizer before dinner if you use expensive beef (then this recipe would serve twelve). To me, there is nothing better than relaxing around a pool on a warm summer evening as the sun sets. This dish makes a perfect accompaniment.

1½ pounds lean beef (top sirloin or tri-tip)
½ cup low-sodium soy sauce
¼ cup fresh lemon juice
1 tablespoon macadamia nut oil
2 tablespoons ground cumin
Salt
Black pepper, freshly ground
24 pearl onions
2 red onions, cut into 12 small pieces
12 mushrooms
12 8-inch bamboo skewers soaked in water

Combine the first nine ingredients in a large bowl, mix well, and marinate for 1 hour at room temperature. Preheat the barbecue. Create your own kabob, threading the beef and mushrooms on a skewer in whatever order you want. You may also add other vegetables as you see appropriate, but be careful not to weigh down the kabobs—this is only lunch or an appetizer. Grill the kabobs until they reach the desired degree of doneness, turning them occasionally. (Cook them about 5 minutes for medium rare.) It is that simple.

Good for A, B, and C dieters.

Barbecued Spareribs

SERVES 6.

What cookbook about a summer resort town is complete without a recipe for spareribs? This healthier version was sent to me by Wanda H. from Kentucky, where they know a thing or two about barbecue. She had lost a total of 47 pounds when she sent me this recipe.

2 tablespoons paprika

1 teaspoon red pepper flakes

2 teaspoons garlic powder

2 teaspoons onion powder

2 teaspoons lo-han, or 2 packets stevia (Lo-han works best in this recipe, as the sauce will need to glaze up.)

1 teaspoon dry mustard powder

1 teaspoon salt

1 teaspoon black pepper, freshly ground

½ teaspoon cayenne pepper

2 tablespoons macadamia nut oil

5 pounds baby back spareribs (I prefer these ribs, but you could also use beef ribs if you like.)

Combine all the ingredients except the oil and the ribs in a small bowl. Place the ribs in a large baking pan or plastic container, and rub down with the oil. Add the dry ingredients, carefully coating the ribs with the mixture. Cover and refrigerate for at least 1 hour but preferably overnight.

When you're ready to cook the ribs, heat the grill and cook over direct heat until the ribs are browned. Then lower the fire, move the ribs to one side of the grill for more indirect heating, and cook for about 45 minutes until there is no pink on the ribs.

Good for A, B, and C dieters.

Cheese and Jalapeño Quesadillas

SERVES 6.

These became one of Jeff's specialties in California while he attended San Diego State University. You can get crazy with the ingredients you add; basically, you can add whatever you want, but remember to stay within the boundaries of your new eating plan. It's so important to have dishes like this, which are so easy to make and yet so versatile. It's one way to ensure that you or your family never gets bored!

2 tablespoons macadamia nut oil
1 red onion, chopped
1 jalapeño, seeded and chopped
1 eggplant, seeded and chopped
Salt
Black pepper, freshly ground
3 tablespoons fresh cilantro, chopped
6 whole wheat tortillas
12 ounces Monterey Jack cheese, grated

Place a medium-size skillet over medium-low heat. Add 1 tablespoon of oil, then the onion, and sauté for 5 minutes or until light brown. Add the jalapeño and eggplant and cook for about 5 more minutes. Remove the contents of the skillet to a large bowl and add the salt, pepper, and cilantro. Mix well and set the bowl aside.

Heat a large skillet over medium-high heat. Add a ½ tablespoon of oil to the skillet, then place a tortilla in the skillet for about 2 minutes, flip it over, and sprinkle 2 ounces of cheese evenly over the tortilla. Top with the onion and jalapeño mixture and cook for about 1 minute until the cheese is melted. Top with another tortilla, then flip it over with a spatula, and cook for about 2 minutes. Slip the quesadilla onto a plate and cut into four sections. Serve hot. Repeat with the remaining tortillas.

Good for A, B, and C dieters.

Summer Squash Soup

SERVES 8.

This is incredibly easy to make and tastes divine. It's especially perfect in the middle of the summer, served cold when squash are at their peak.

¼ cup macadamia nut oil
8 cups yellow squash, diced
4 stalks celery, with leaves, diced
1 medium onion, diced
64 ounces organic chicken broth or homemade
    organic chicken stock
1 pint heavy cream
½ cup Parmesan cheese
Black pepper, freshly ground
Salt, to taste

Over medium heat, add the macadamia nut oil to a large soup pot. Add the squash, celery, and onion. Cover and cook until the vegetables are soft and the squash starts to break down. Add the chicken broth and simmer until the broth reduces by half. Add the heavy cream and Parmesan cheese and mix thoroughly. Just before serving, add pepper, and taste the soup to see if it needs any salt.

This may be served with a small dollop of sour cream or a pinch of cayenne pepper.

Good for A, B, and C dieters.

Lentil Soup

Lentils are a versatile legume that can be enjoyed as a soup, a salad, or an accompaniment to fish or meat. Many different kinds are grown throughout the world and have entered into most countries' gastronomic histories—especially countries along the Mediterranean coast. They are also a good source of protein for vegetarians. What makes them part of the Hamptons Diet is their role in how they affect blood sugar. They have a low glycemic index, and this recipe has a very low glycemic load, making it a perfect meal for a cool, crisp fall day or a cold winter evening. You can lose weight eating lentils—it all depends on the serving size.

1 cup brown or green lentils
3 cups chicken stock
1 onion, minced
1 carrot, minced
1 celery stalk, minced
1 garlic clove, minced
1 leek, minced
1 tomato, skinned, seeded, and chopped
1 bay leaf
1 teaspoon fresh thyme, chopped
1 teaspoon smoked paprika
¼ teaspoon red pepper flakes
4 ounces smoked bacon, uncured and nitrate-free
4 ounces chorizo sausage, quartered
2 tablespoons macadamia nut oil
Salt
Black pepper, freshly ground

Rinse the lentils under cold water. Add the chicken stock and lentils to a 6-quart pot and place it over medium heat. Bring to a soft boil and skim off the brownish scum that rises to the top.

Add the next thirteen ingredients. Let the soup simmer for about 45 minutes or until the lentils are soft. Add salt and pepper to taste. Serve hot.

Good for B and C dieters.

Lentil Soup, Mama Pescatore Variation

Being Italian, my mother used to prepare this soup in a similar fashion, only at the end she added a 16-ounce box of pasta and 16 ounces more of water for a very hearty soup. I recommend that you use only a whole-grain pasta if you choose to try the dish this way.

For people who are on the B or the C phase of this diet program, there is nothing wrong with whole-grain pasta. Whole grain is healthy, provided that the ingredient list specifies the word whole. *Whole-grain pasta comes in wheat, buckwheat, spelt, kamut, quinoa, amaranth, brown rice, and other varieties. Just be sure to cook it al dente, and your family or friends won't know the difference.*

Good for C dieters.

Gazpacho Andalucia

SERVES 8.

This soup is one of Spain's most popular dishes. It is very healthy and flavorful. You should let it sit in the refrigerator overnight so that all the flavors combine and come to life. It may be served cold or heated; Jeff has served this as a sauce over fresh fish that were caught that day in the Mediterranean Sea.

¼ pound day-old whole-grain spelt bread
½ cup cold water
1 cucumber, peeled and seeded
½ red bell pepper, cored and seeded
½ green bell pepper, cored and seeded
2 cloves garlic
¼ cup sherry vinegar
2 drops Tabasco sauce
1 teaspoon lo-han or 2 packets stevia
1 teaspoon salt
6 ripe tomatoes, peeled, seeded, and cut up
½ cup macadamia nut oil

If you want to make extra thick soup, soak the bread in water for about 5 minutes. This is an optional step. I have made this recipe without the bread, and it tastes equally delicious. If you desire an even thicker consistency, add some of the pureed cauliflower found in the Whipped Mock Potatoes recipe on page 176.

In a blender or a food processor, add all of the ingredients except the oil and bread, and blend for several minutes until well mixed. Add the bread and pulse for a few more minutes. Then, with the blender still running, slowly add the oil. Check the seasonings and correct as needed. Put the soup in a glass bowl, cover, and refrigerate overnight.

If bread is used, good for B and C dieters. If bread is not used, good for A, B, and C dieters.

Quick and Easy Chicken Rice Soup

SERVES 6.

This soup is quick and easy, but it's also very tasty, especially on a cold winter day or when you are feeling a bit under the weather. We have yet to figure out why chicken soup is so universally recommended for someone who has a cold or the flu, but there is scientific evidence to support its use, so make a big batch, divide it into smaller portions, stick it in the freezer, and defrost it at will. It won't go bad, and then you'll always have it.

1 cup chicken, finely chopped
2 tablespoons butter
¼ cup whole wheat flour
3 small chicken stock cubes, crumbled
3½ cups hot water
⅓ cup brown rice
2½ tablespoons lemon juice
½ tablespoon fresh tarragon leaves
Salt
Black pepper, freshly ground

In a large stock pot, bring salted water to a rolling boil. Add the chicken and heat for about 30 to 45 minutes until it's fully cooked. Drain and set aside the chicken. Heat the butter in the stock pan over medium heat until melted. Add the flour, stirring until it starts to bubble. Stir in the stock cubes and 3½ cups of water. Stir over the heat until the mixture boils. Add the remaining ingredients and the cooked chicken and simmer until the rice is done, about 20 minutes. Add salt and pepper to taste.

Good for B and C dieters.

Bibb Lettuce with Duck Confit and Toasted Almonds

SERVES 4.

Salads are one of my favorite lunchtime meals. As I've said, I usually eat a salad in-between patients at the office. Salads are easy to prepare and are one of those dishes that is limited only by whatever ingredients are available. The Hamptons rule of fresh, local, and seasonal always applies to salads. Salads make great side dishes, as well as delicious dinners.

The trick to cooking Hamptons Diet–style is to learn the basics and then be creative with the ingredients. Never be tied down to what the recipe recommends. Once you know how to mix lettuces, the salad ingredients can be mixed in any way, shape, or form. For health reasons, I usually try to add as many different colors of ingredients as I can find. In this way, you get the most antioxidants and bioflavonoids from your meal. Salads are another "kitchen-sink" dish in my household. Whatever is in the refrigerator gets thrown on top of a bed of lettuce with some healthful dressing.

Jeff came up with some great lunch salads for this chapter and also some tasty side salads that you will find in chapter 6.

Jeff's love affair with duck confit began when he lived in France; confit is found everywhere there and is used in many different recipes. For people who are not familiar with confit, it is simply duck meat that has been wrapped and cooked in its own fat. I find duck confit to be absolutely delicious, sweet, and juicy. It transforms a salad into a meal.

The first time I had duck confit was at a Bastille Day celebration in a little restaurant called Florent in the meat-packing district of New York City. This was about fifteen years ago when that neighborhood had just one restaurant and quite a few transvestite hookers—pretty colorful, huh? Every July 14, the restaurant hosted a big block party, and it seemed as if the entire city showed up and partied 'til the wee hours. The party still happens, the neighborhood is now very trendy, and I'm too old to party like that—but this duck confit recipe is a classic and tastes as good as my first one.

Bibb Lettuce with Duck Confit and Toasted Almonds (*continued*)

    1 duck thigh confit (can be bought at a good butcher shop)
    2 ounces almonds, sliced, blanched
    2 tablespoons sherry vinegar
    3 tablespoons macadamia nut oil
    3 tablespoons extra-virgin olive oil
    Salt
    Black pepper, freshly ground
    2 heads Bibb lettuce, washed and dried

Heat a small skillet over medium heat. Add the confit and cook for about 5 minutes until light brown. Turn it and cook for another 5 minutes. Remove the thigh from the heat and let it cool slightly. When it's cool enough to handle, take the meat off the bone and return the meat to the skillet, along with the almonds. Cook until the almonds are toasted, about 3 minutes. Strain the duck and almonds, and place them on a paper towel.

Meanwhile, in a large bowl add the vinegar, oils, and salt and pepper and mix well with a wire whisk. Add the dried lettuce leaves to this mixture and toss well. Divide the salad onto 4 plates and top each plate with the duck meat and almonds.

As a variation, you can use tuna, salmon, or sliced steak.

Good for A, B, and C dieters.

5

Hamptons Diet
Dinner Recipes

Although it may be impossible to get a reservation at your favorite restaurant in the Hamptons unless you have a famous name, this doesn't mean that dinner can't be one of the most enjoyable and entertaining parts of the day. In fact, it's my favorite time of the day. Work is over, and it's time for friends and family. Many of the recipes in this section can be used for entertaining, although there is also a separate chapter for those occasions. The thing I like most about these recipes is that when you make them, there is always enough for leftovers, which means lunch and breakfast.

Broccoli Cheese Soup

SERVES 6–8.

Broccoli is available year-round, but it's really popular in the fall and the winter when other vegetables aren't in season. Jeff visited Switzerland several times while living in France, and each time he had traditional fondue made of Gruyère and Emmental cheeses. These cheeses are used because of their excellent melting properties, creaminess, and wonderful flavor. If you use these two cheeses, your guests will be blown away. If you can't find these cheeses, then a good mild cheddar will work.

4 cups broccoli florets, chopped (plus extra for optional garnish)
1 cup Spanish onion, chopped
1 clove garlic, minced
1 large celery root, peeled and sliced
1 cup chicken stock
1 bay leaf
1¾ cups heavy cream
¾ cup Gruyère cheese
¾ cup Emmental cheese
¼ teaspoon Madras curry powder
Pinch cayenne pepper
Salt
White pepper, freshly ground
Chives, optional garnish
Sour cream, optional garnish

In a medium saucepan over medium heat, combine the broccoli, onion, garlic, celery root, stock, and bay leaf. Bring to a boil. Reduce the heat to medium-low and simmer, covered, until the vegetables are tender, about 15 minutes. Discard the bay leaf. Transfer the mixture to a blender and puree in as many batches as are needed. Return the mixture to the pan and add the remaining ingredients. Slowly bring the soup to a simmer, stirring until the cheese melts. Serve the soup in bowls. Save some of the broccoli florets as a garnish if you like or sprinkle chopped chives onto the soup and top with a dollop of sour cream.

Good for A, B, and C dieters.

Roasted Tomato and Onion Soup with Fresh Herbs

SERVES 8.

Jeff grew to love slow roasting when he lived in Spain. He tells me that many foods are slow roasted there, probably because no one ever seems to be in a rush. At Candido, in Segovia, about an hour's drive north of Madrid, he used to slow roast lamb and suckling pig. Because they had a huge brick oven going all day, they often found other things to roast, such as tomatoes and onions. By roasting these two vegetables, you add a slight smoky flavor to dishes you use them in.

10 (about 2 pounds) ripe fresh tomatoes, halved crosswise
2 Spanish onions, peeled and quartered
Kosher salt
Black pepper, freshly ground
¼ cup macadamia nut oil
2 cloves garlic, minced
2 tablespoons fresh basil, chopped
2 tablespoons fresh rosemary, chopped
2 tablespoons fresh thyme, chopped
4 cups chicken stock
¼ cup dry red wine
½ cup heavy cream
3 tablespoons Parmesan cheese, grated

Preheat the oven to 375°F. Place the tomatoes cut-side up in a lightly oiled glass baking dish. Add the onions. Season the tomatoes and onions with salt and pepper. In a small bowl, mix the oil, garlic, and herbs. Spread this mixture evenly over the tomatoes and onions. Roast until the tomatoes are soft and lightly browned, about 45 minutes. Scrape the tomatoes, onions, and juices into a food processor and puree until smooth.

Transfer the pureed mixture to a soup pot over medium heat. Add the remaining ingredients and simmer, uncovered, 15 to 20 minutes. Add more salt and pepper if needed.

Good for B and C dieters.

Creamy Chickpea and Farro Soup

SERVES 6–8.

Jeff first learned of farro when he was working at Il Buco in New York City, which received this grain directly from Italy. Farro has a complex nutty taste and is more elegant than most whole wheat grains. You can substitute hulled barley if you like; just don't soak it overnight.

1 cup dried chickpeas
1 cup farro or hulled barley
1 medium Spanish onion, quartered
1 medium carrot, peeled and quartered
1 teaspoon sea salt
2 bay leaves
¼ cup macadamia nut oil
1 large Spanish onion, chopped
1 tablespoon prosciutto, chopped
2 tablespoons celery, chopped
1½ quarts chicken stock
1 teaspoon dried marjoram
Pinch nutmeg, freshly grated
Black pepper, freshly ground
Flat-leaf parsley, freshly chopped, for garnish

Rinse the chickpeas and soak them overnight in enough cold water to cover them. Do the same with the farro, separately.

Drain the chickpeas and place them in a large soup pot. Cover them with cold water and bring to a boil over medium heat. Spoon out any foam that rises to the surface. Add the quartered onion and carrot. Then add the salt and bay leaves. Reduce the heat to low and simmer, partially covered, until the chickpeas are very soft, about 1½ hours.

Meanwhile, in a medium saucepan, heat 2 tablespoons of macadamia nut oil over medium-low heat and gently cook the onion, prosciutto, and celery for 5 to 6 minutes, stirring occasionally, until they are soft but not brown. Drain the farro and add it, along with the stock and marjoram, to the onions and cook, partially covered, for about 1 hour.

Drain the chickpeas, reserving the cooking liquid, and discard the bay leaves. Puree the chickpeas with 1½ cups of the reserved cooking liquid, the onion, and the carrot in a food processor. Add the pureed mixture to the farro and, if necessary, add more of the chickpeas' cooking liquid to achieve a creamy consistency. Add a pinch of nutmeg, some freshly ground pepper, and salt if needed. Pour into soup bowls and sprinkle with parsley. Finish with a drizzle of macadamia nut oil.

Good for B and C dieters.

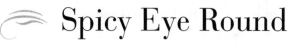

Spicy Eye Round

SERVES 10.

Eye round is one of my favorite cuts of meat. This recipe, sent to me from Georgia W., inspires me to make it each time I think about it. Guests simply love this dish.

1 5-pound eye round roast
3 onions, sliced
½ teaspoon salt
¼ teaspoon black pepper, freshly ground
Spicy Sauce (recipe follows)

Preheat the oven to 350°F.

Place the roast in a roasting pan and add the onions, salt, and pepper. Bake uncovered for 3½ hours. Cool the roast and cut into thin slices, then place them in a large ovenproof container. Add the Spicy Sauce, cover, and chill for 8 hours. Remove the roast from the refrigerator and let stand at room temperature for 30 minutes. Bake again in a 350°F oven for 45 minutes or until it reaches your desired degree of doneness.

Spicy Sauce

MAKES 7 CUPS.

2 cups water
2 fresh tomatoes, diced
2 large onions, sliced
⅓ cup red wine vinegar
2 tablespoons Worcestershire sauce
1 teaspoon mustard powder
1 teaspoon dried oregano
1 teaspoon black pepper, freshly ground
1 teaspoon garlic powder
½ teaspoon chili powder

½ teaspoon cloves, ground
¼ teaspoon nutmeg, ground
½ teaspoon Tabasco sauce
1 bay leaf

Bring all the ingredients to a boil in a Dutch oven over medium heat. Reduce the heat to low and cook for 1 hour. Cool the sauce and discard the bay leaf.

Good for A, B, and C dieters.

rilled Skirt Steak
ith Chimichurri

SERVES 4.

This recipe was sent to me by a reader from Los Gatos, California. The skirt steak is a nice, inexpensive cut of meat and is affordable for most budgets. The members of this family didn't need to lose any weight but simply followed the Hamptons Diet approach for health reasons. Here is their recipe. This makes a great early summer barbecue idea when the evenings are still cool. The spices will be sure to heat you up.

1 Thai chili (or any hot chili like habanero—for a milder version, use jalapeño)
2 large shallots, chopped
½ cup fresh mint, chopped
½ cup fresh cilantro, chopped
3 cloves garlic, chopped
2 tablespoons fresh lime juice
Black pepper, coarsely ground
1½ pounds skirt steak
16 Boston lettuce leaves
1 tablespoon Thai fish sauce (found in any ethnic grocery store)

Heat a gas grill with a medium-hot fire. Combine all the ingredients except the steak and lettuce in a food processor and pulse—do not puree. Season the steak with salt and pepper and grill for 4 minutes on each side for medium rare—longer according to individual preferences. Remove the steak from the heat, cut into strips, and arrange over the lettuce. Add the sauce, roll up, and serve.

Good for A, B, and C dieters.

Garlic Rosemary Chicken

SERVES 4–6.

This recipe was sent to me by one of my favorite patients, Irene K. She always brings me fresh, organic vegetables from her garden—especially home-grown peppers, which she knows I love. They are the best peppers I've ever eaten in my life. This recipe reminds me of home.

6 chicken thighs or breasts
Salt
Black pepper, freshly ground
2 teaspoons fresh basil, chopped
1 teaspoon dried oregano
20 garlic cloves, peeled and left whole
½ cup dry white wine
1 cup macadamia nut oil
4 celery ribs, thickly sliced about 1 inch thick
4 carrots, sliced into ½-inch sections
3 leeks, white parts only, sliced
4 sprigs fresh rosemary, torn into hearty pieces
Juice of 1 lemon

Preheat the oven to 375°F.

Place the chicken pieces skin-side up in a baking pan. Season with salt, pepper, fresh basil, and dried oregano. Combine the garlic, wine, oil, celery, carrots, leeks, and rosemary in a mixing bowl and stir thoroughly. Pour this mixture and the lemon juice over the chicken, then run your hands over the chicken to coat all the pieces evenly. Cover the chicken and pan with aluminum foil and bake for 40 minutes. Remove the foil and bake the chicken for an additional 15 minutes.

Good for A, B, and C dieters.

Garlic and Lemon Chicken

SERVES 10–12.

Pollo al ajillo, garlic chicken, is one of Spain's most popular dishes, simple and tasty. Here is Jeff's rendition of this classic.

4 large chicken breasts, skinless and boneless
¼ cup macadamia nut oil
Salt
Black pepper, freshly ground
1 Spanish onion, finely chopped
8 garlic cloves, finely sliced
2 lemons, zest of 1 and juice of both
½ cup flat-leaf parsley, chopped
Lemon wedges for garnish

Slice each chicken breast into long, thin slices. Heat the oil in a large, thick-bottomed skillet over medium-high heat. Salt and pepper the chicken strips and place in the skillet. Cook until lightly browned, about 7 to 8 minutes. Remove the chicken from the skillet and lower the heat to medium-low. Add the onion and cook for about 5 minutes, stirring frequently, until softened but not browned. Add the garlic and cook for another 2 minutes. Add the lemon juice and zest and deglaze the skillet by scraping and stirring all the bits on the bottom of the skillet with a wooden spoon. Place the chicken strips back into the skillet. Sprinkle with the parsley and toss well to coat the chicken with the sauce. Put the hot chicken on a warm serving plate and garnish with lemon wedges.

Good for A, B, and C dieters.

Grilled Baby Chicken Al Mattone

SERVES 6–8.

When Jeff worked in Italy, Sunday was his day off. So on Sundays, he and his coworkers often took a bus up to a nearby lake, where the Italians he worked with grilled baby chickens. The only thing they did differently when grilling was to place a brick on top of each chicken to weigh it down. This created a nice crispy skin. Jeff has used this technique ever since he left Italy.

I tried to do this once when making pizza, using bricks that are supposed to heat things evenly. I was staying at a friend's home in upstate New York and, to make a very long story short, I ended up burning the bricks, setting off the smoke alarms, and having to answer to a small town's fire department. As my friend was a national news anchor, this was in all the newspapers, and she didn't find it nearly as amusing as I did. Here's hoping you will have more success than I did with this technique.

2 whole baby chickens, backbone removed, flattened
Salt
Black pepper, freshly ground
¼ cup macadamia nut oil
2 bricks wrapped in foil

Rinse the chickens and pat dry. Season with salt and pepper and set aside. Prepare a very hot grill or heat the oil in a cast-iron skillet over high heat, allowing it to get very hot—almost to the smoke point. Place the chickens on the grill or in the skillet and weigh them down with the bricks. Cook over high heat, turning about every 3 minutes, for a total of 15 minutes, or until they are crispy and cooked through. Jeff likes to serve this chicken over summer greens, such as the ensalada mixta in the side dish chapter.

Good for A, B, and C dieters.

Mediterranean Roast Chicken

SERVES 6–8.

Chef Jeff tells us, "Several years ago I was riding my bike through the vineyards of Catalonia just outside of Barcelona and came upon an incredible barbecue smell, unlike anything I had experienced before. I turned the corner and saw the smoke rising from a tiny roadside wooden shack. Inside the shack they were roasting the chickens whole. Even though I was riding alone, I had to order a whole bird just to find out what made this incredible aroma and hopefully incredible taste. They packed up a chicken, and I rode down the road a bit, pulled over, and ate the best chicken of my life." Here is that recipe, updated.

1 3- or 3½-pound roasting chicken
Kosher salt
Black pepper, freshly ground
1 cup fresh herbs (thyme, rosemary, parsley, marjoram, sage), chopped
2 bay leaves
1 lemon, quartered
1 head garlic, halved
3 tablespoons macadamia nut oil

Preheat the oven to 425°F. Wash the chicken inside and out and pat it as dry as you can with paper towels. Rub the cavity with salt and pepper, then fill the cavity with all the ingredients except for the oil. Rub the chicken with the oil. Place the chicken in a roasting pan and put in the oven for 15 minutes. Then turn down the oven to 350°F and cook for 45 minutes longer. Remove the chicken from the oven and let it sit for 10 minutes before carving it.

Good for A, B, and C dieters.

Prosciutto- and Provolone- Stuffed Chicken Breasts

SERVES 8.

This takes the place of traditional Italian chicken cutlets. Okay, maybe not completely, but the dish is certainly a close second and one you will absolutely enjoy.

Macadamia nut oil
4 chicken breast halves, boneless, skinless, trimmed of fat
    and cartilage if necessary
4 slices provolone cheese, cut in half
4 slices prosciutto
4 teaspoons stoneground mustard
4 large fresh basil leaves
Garlic powder
Italian herb seasoning
Black pepper, coarsely ground

Grease a 9- × 11-inch baking dish with 2 teaspoons of macadamia nut oil and preheat the oven to 350°F. Pound each chicken breast between two pieces of plastic wrap until thin and flat. On each breast, put two cheese halves (down the center in a line) and one slice of prosciutto. Smear 1 teaspoon of the mustard on the prosciutto. Place a basil leaf on top of the mustard. Roll the chicken breasts up and lay them seam-side down in the baking dish.

Drizzle macadamia nut oil on the breast rolls. Sprinkle them to taste with garlic powder, Italian herb seasoning, and black pepper. Cover with foil and bake for about 35 minutes or until they're no longer pink. Remove the foil and put the breasts under the broiler until the tops are slightly golden.

Place the chicken on plates and drizzle the juice from the baking dish over them.

Good for A, B, and C dieters.

Almond Dijon Baked Chicken

SERVES 4.

When Jeff lived in Lyon, France, his friend's mother used to make this dish all the time. It is very French and very easy. There are only a few ingredients, so even the most finicky person can enjoy this.

4 chicken breasts, boneless, skinless
Macadamia nut oil in a spray bottle
Salt
Black pepper, freshly ground
2 tablespoons Dijon mustard
½ cup raw almonds, sliced (chopped is fine)

Preheat the oven to 350°F.

Place the chicken in a baking pan sprayed with oil. Lightly salt and pepper the chicken. Then spread the mustard on top of the chicken and sprinkle it with the almonds. Bake for about 20 minutes or until the chicken is done. If the almonds start to get too brown, place aluminum foil over the chicken.

Good for A, B, and C dieters.

Baked Cod with Orange-Saffron Cream Sauce

SERVES 4.

Cod is a deliciously mild, white, flaky fish that is at its best in the fall. Jeff created this dish while cooking for a famous New York fashion designer. Designers like to stay as trim as their models, so fish dishes are popular with that crowd. This recipe makes a delicious and filling main course either for your family or to impress your friends. Steamed broccoli would be a nice accompaniment for this dish.

2 tablespoons avocado oil
1½ pounds fresh cod fillets
Juice of ½ orange
¼ cup white wine
2 tablespoons champagne vinegar
½ teaspoon saffron
1 cup heavy cream
Salt
White pepper, freshly ground

Heat the 2 tablespoons of oil in a 16-inch nonstick skillet over medium-high heat. When the oil is almost smoking, gently lay the fillets in the skillet. Cook for 7 to 8 minutes without turning the fillets over. Using a spatula, carefully remove the fillets, place on a plate, and cover with aluminum foil.

Lower the heat to medium. Add the orange juice, white wine, champagne vinegar, and saffron. Reduce this mixture until there are only about 2 tablespoons of liquid left. Add the heavy cream and reduce the liquid by half. Add salt and pepper to taste. Divide the cod onto 4 plates and pour the sauce over the fish.

Good for A, B, and C dieters.

acadamia Coconut Salmon

s 4.

The next recipe (and three others in this book) came from a Hamptons Diet recipe contest sponsored by my good friends at www.trulylowcarb.com.

I chose this recipe to be one of the finalists because it combines many healthy aspects of cooking in the Hamptons Diet style: wild fish, macadamia nut oil, and fresh ingredients.

4–5 tablespoons macadamia nut oil
¼ cup macadamia nuts, crushed, unsalted
¼ cup coconut flakes, unsweetened
1 tablespoon garlic, minced
1 teaspoon sea salt
1 teaspoon black pepper, freshly ground
4 salmon fillets (wild Alaskan, if possible), skin removed
4 slices lemon

Preheat the oven to 350°F.

On the stove heat 2 tablespoons of macadamia nut oil to a medium temperature in an ovenproof pan. In a bowl, combine the macadamia nuts, coconut, garlic, salt, and pepper. Rub 1 tablespoon of oil onto the salmon fillets, then press the dry ingredients onto both sides of the salmon. Sauté one side of the salmon fillets in oil. Flip them over in the pan and then put the pan in the oven. For rare, 3 to 4 minutes is all it takes. For more well-done fillets, leave in the oven for 10 minutes. Garnish with lemon and more oil as needed.

Good for A, B, and C dieters.

- note - even for medium need to cook longer. like 25 minutes baking at 400° with a good thick cut. or sear longer on both sides (like 3-4 mins/side) before baking

- 2.15/05/17 - correct 350° for 20 mins good (sear 2 mins/ side on pan)

Salmon with Baby Spinach

SERVES 4.

This recipe was sent to me by one of my friends in Thailand. People who know me know that I travel through Asia quite a bit and have been able to pick up many recipe ideas and tricks from those places. I have found that the food never tastes quite the same over here because we just don't have access to the same spices, which is what Asian food is all about. This recipe comes very close, though.

6 tablespoons macadamia nut oil

3 tablespoons lemongrass, chopped, without root ends
   or dried tops

2 cloves garlic, minced

2 tablespoons fresh turmeric, chopped (it's okay to use
   ground if fresh is unavailable)

1 teaspoon of coriander seeds, toasted, ground

1 teaspoon chili paste

3 tablespoons shallots, minced

1 cup heavy cream

Salt

Black pepper, freshly ground

4 6-ounce salmon fillets, with skin

2 cups baby spinach, chopped small but not minced

Nutmeg, freshly ground (optional)

Preheat the oven to 450°F.

Put half of the macadamia nut oil into a small saucepan over medium heat. Add the lemongrass, garlic, turmeric, coriander, chili paste, and shallots. Stir until the mixture is fragrant and golden brown. Add the cream and ½ cup of water and simmer for 3 minutes. Strain and season with salt and pepper to taste. Set it aside and keep warm.

Season the salmon with salt and pepper. Put 1 tablespoon of the oil in a large nonstick skillet over low heat. When the oil is hot, add the salmon, skin-side down, and allow it to cook until the skin is crisp, about 3 minutes. Remove from the heat, set aside, and keep warm.

In a sauté pan over medium-high heat, add the remaining oil. When the oil is hot, add the remaining shallots and sauté until brown. Add the spinach and sauté for 1 minute. Divide the spinach evenly among four plates and arrange the salmon on top. Spoon the sauce over the salmon. You may want to sprinkle some freshly ground nutmeg on top before serving it.

Good for A, B, and C dieters.

Halibut in Parchment Paper with Fennel and Grapefruit

SERVES 4.

While working in northern Italy, Jeff learned about cooking in cartoccio, *or parchment paper. He often used a Mediterranean fish that is similar to halibut. That's where he first cooked with this fennel and grapefruit combination, which he's subsequently used in other dishes because of the amazing flavor combination. Cooking in parchment paper is an excellent way to retain moisture and flavor.*

4 6-ounce halibut fillets, boneless, skinless
Salt
White pepper, freshly ground
4 tablespoons macadamia nut oil
1 large grapefruit, cut into segments, with no pith attached
1 tablespoon fennel seeds
1 fennel bulb, cut in half and very thinly sliced
½ cup dry white wine

Preheat the oven to 450°F.

Season the fish fillets with salt and pepper. Cut parchment paper into four 24- × 48-inch pieces. Drizzle 1 tablespoon of the oil in the center of each piece and top it with a quarter of the grapefruit, fennel seeds, and fennel bulb. Lay a halibut fillet over the grapefruit and fennel. Drizzle 2 tablespoons of wine over each fillet. Fold the paper up around the ingredients to form a packet.

Place the packets on a sheet pan and bake in the oven for 15 minutes. Remove the packets from the oven and slice the paper with a knife, taking care to avoid burning yourself with the steam. Serve immediately.

Good for A, B, and C dieters.

Baked Fish Fillets with Lemon and Capers

SERVES 4.

4 fish fillets (about 8 ounces each), any kind, boneless, skinless
Salt
Black pepper, freshly ground
⅓ cup macadamia nut oil
2 cloves garlic, thinly sliced
2 tablespoons tarragon, chopped
1 lemon, carved with a knife into segments
3 tablespoons capers
2 tablespoons chives, chopped
¼ cup dry white wine
¼ cup clam juice, bottled

Preheat oven to 325°F.

Line a sheet pan with aluminum foil with enough foil overhanging to later cover the fish. Season the fish fillets with salt and pepper and drizzle the macadamia nut oil onto the foil covering the bottom of the pan. Place the fillets on top of the oil and curl the edges of the foil up, creating a lip to prevent the liquids from escaping. Sprinkle the remaining ingredients over the fillets, cover with the other half of the aluminum foil, and bake for 20 minutes or until cooked through, depending on the thickness of the fillets. Garnish with lemon segments.

Good for A, B, and C dieters.

Steamed Shrimp and New Zealand Cockles

SERVES 4–6.

Jeff tells us that the Spanish consume the second-largest amount of seafood, per person, in the world. Two of their favorites are shrimp and clams. This is a dish with several flavors you wouldn't traditionally find in Spain. If you can't find New Zealand cockles, use littleneck clams.

½ cup macadamia nut oil
5 garlic cloves, peeled and minced
1 cup dry white wine
25–30 New Zealand cockles
12 gulf shrimp, peeled and deveined
1 jalapeño, seeded and finely chopped
Handful fresh parsley, chopped
Handful fresh basil leaves, finely shredded

In a deep, large skillet or a stock pot, heat 2 tablespoons of the oil until very hot but not smoking. Add the garlic and cook for 1 to 2 minutes, until very lightly browned. Add the wine, cockles, shrimp, and jalapeño and cover. Lower the heat to medium and cook for 3 to 4 minutes. The clams should open, and the shrimp should be cooked through. Discard any unopened clams.

Add the parsley and toss the seafood gently over low heat for about 1 minute, then remove from the heat. Add the remaining oil and mix well. Divide the seafood among four warm bowls and sprinkle with the basil. Serve immediately.

Good for A, B, and C dieters.

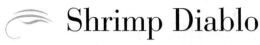

Shrimp Diablo

SERVES 4.

Diablo *means "devil" in Spanish—and you'll feel like a devil because you won't want to share this delicious recipe with anyone. It's a little spicy but not so much that it will turn someone off to this dish.*

½ cup chili sauce, unsweetened, from a Thai or other
    specialty grocery store
2 teaspoons fresh lime juice
1 teaspoon white horseradish (creamy)
¼ teaspoon Tabasco sauce
Salt
Black pepper, freshly ground
1 pound large shrimp, cooked and peeled

Combine all the ingredients, except the shrimp, in a bowl. Mix well and refrigerate for 15 minutes before serving. Plate the shrimp and serve the sauce on the side.

Good for A, B, and C dieters.

Udon Noodles Alfredo with Peas and Ham

SERVES 8.

Udon is not the Philadelphia way of saying "Hold on." Udon is a type of noodle from Asia that is extremely healthy; it is made from whole grain and is therefore encouraged on the Hamptons Diet. This recipe is a variation of the old Italian classic Fettuccine Alfredo. Kids love this dish because of the sauce, and they never even realize that they aren't eating white pasta. Your husband and guests will love it, too. My patients have used this recipe for their kids' sleepovers with friends. They never knew the difference and wanted to know why it tasted so good.

1 16-ounce package udon noodles
1 tablespoon macadamia nut oil
1 small onion, chopped
1 clove garlic, minced
½ cup diced ham (sugar-free and nitrate-free, if possible)
1 bay leaf
2 cups heavy cream
3 tablespoons Parmesan cheese, grated, plus extra for optional garnish
½ cup peas
Salt
White pepper, freshly ground
Pinch nutmeg, freshly ground
1 egg yolk

Bring 2 quarts of salted water to a rapid boil. Add the noodles and cook for 8 to 10 minutes or until done. Strain and rinse under cold water.

Heat 1 tablespoon of macadamia nut oil over medium-low heat in a medium saucepan. Add the onion and sauté for 5 minutes until translucent. Add the garlic and ham and cook for 2 minutes. Add the bay leaf, cream, and Parmesan cheese. Cook over low heat for about 15 minutes until slightly thick. Discard the bay leaf. Add the peas, salt, pepper, and nutmeg. Remove from the heat, let cool slightly, and whisk in the egg yolk. Mix the noodles into the sauce well. Serve the noodles in bowls and top with grated Parmesan if desired.

Good for B and C dieters.

Sausage, Bacon, and Bean Casserole

SERVES 6–8.

Legumes are an essential part of the Mediterranean diet and the Hamptons Diet. Slowly cooked, they become filled with flavor and have a soft, creamy texture. This casserole is perfect for a cold winter night. There are so many different kinds of sausage on the market; choose the one you like best. Feel free to use chicken sausage if you prefer. My only advice is to choose a type that is nitrate-free.

1½ cups dried cannellini beans
2 tablespoons avocado oil
8 slices smoked lean bacon, nitrate-free and not sugar-cured
8 medium pork sausages (not sugar-cured)
3 large carrots, chopped
3 large onions, chopped
2 celery sticks, chopped
2 garlic cloves
2 bay leaves
2 fresh thyme sprigs
3 cups chicken stock
Salt
Black pepper, freshly ground

Put the beans in a large pot, cover with cold water, and let them sit overnight. The next morning drain the beans.

When you're ready to cook this dish, preheat the oven to 300°F. Put all the ingredients, except for salt and pepper, in a large, flameproof casserole dish. Bring the mixture to a soft boil over medium heat. Cover the dish and bake for 3 to 4 hours, stirring occasionally and topping off the liquid if necessary. You want the beans to be soft and creamy but not falling apart. Take the casserole out of the oven. Discard the bay leaves and thyme sprigs. Let the casserole sit for 15 minutes before serving.

Good for B and C dieters.

Stuffed Pork Chops with Spinach, Cheese, and Pine Nuts

SERVES 4.

Jeff recommends that you ask your butcher for the rib chops, as they are the best for stuffing. Jeff also suggests that the key to good stuffed pork chops is not to use a dry stuffing. I love pork chops, and I especially love them when they are stuffed.

4 bone-in pork rib chops, 1½ inches thick
1 tablespoon macadamia nut oil
Salt
Black pepper, freshly ground
Spinach, Cheese, and Pine Nut Stuffing (recipe follows)

Preheat the oven to 450°F.

Insert a sharp paring knife through the side of each chop until it touches the bone. The opening should be only about 1 inch. Now move the knife back and forth in opposite directions, making a pocket as large as possible while keeping the opening as small as possible. Fill the chops with the stuffing using your thumb and index finger. Top each hole with a lemon wedge.

Heat the oil in a heavy-bottomed ovenproof skillet over medium-high heat until the oil just begins to smoke. Season the chops with salt and pepper and place in the skillet. Cook for 3 minutes on one side, flip them over and then place the skillet into the oven. Cook the chops for about 15 minutes, turning them over halfway through. Take them out, transfer to a plate, and cover with foil. Let them sit for 10 minutes before serving.

Spinach, Cheese, and Pine Nut Stuffing
MAKES 2 CUPS.

This stuffing can be used for roasting chickens, turkeys, and even breast of lamb. The stuffing is universal, and the meat is the part that changes in this recipe. Don't be afraid to try this with different cuts of meat that look interesting or that are organic on sale that day at the butcher's. Again, each variation is like a clean slate, with the stuffing being the texture.

¼ cup pine nuts, toasted
1 slice whole-grain bread, torn into pieces
1 tablespoon macadamia nut oil
1 garlic clove, minced
10 cups spinach leaves, washed
1 cup fontina cheese, grated
¼ cup ricotta cheese
¼ cup Parmesan cheese, grated
Salt and pepper
Pinch nutmeg
1 lemon, quartered

To toast the pine nuts, place them on a cookie sheet in a 400°F oven for 5 minutes, or heat them in a skillet until they just start to get brown. Don't over-cook them, or they will get soggy. In a food processor, pulse the bread and toasted pine nuts until well ground.

Heat the oil in a skillet over medium heat, add the garlic, and cook for about 1 minute. Add the spinach and mix well until it's wilted. Place the spinach in a strainer and press out the excess moisture.

In a mixing bowl, add the cheeses and stir them together. Add the breadcrumb–pine nut mixture and the spinach and mix well. Stir in the salt, pepper, and nutmeg.

Good for A, B, and C dieters.

Oven-Roasted Vegetables with Pork

SERVES 8.

Lonny F. sent me this recipe from California. He uses only farm-fresh ingredients and has been thrilled with the variety of food on the Hamptons Diet program. He and his wife have lost a combined weight of 68 pounds.

1½ pounds pork tenderloin, boneless
Macadamia nut oil in a spray bottle
1 medium onion, cut into wedges
2 stalks celery, thinly sliced
2 Japanese eggplants, cut into 1-inch cubes
1 tablespoon macadamia nut oil
2 tablespoons fresh rosemary, crushed
1 tablespoon dried sage, crushed
¼ teaspoon salt
¼ teaspoon black pepper, freshly ground

Preheat the oven to 450°F.

Brown the pork in a skillet sprayed with macadamia nut oil over medium-high heat. Place the pork in a sprayed roasting pan. Arrange the vegetables around the pork and drizzle with macadamia nut oil. Sprinkle the rosemary and other spices evenly over the pork. Bake for 30 minutes until the vegetables are tender, stirring occasionally.

Good for A, B, and C dieters.

Double Pork Chop with Lemon and Thyme

Serves 4.

Pork is eaten in Europe and in the United States, but the cuts are different. The double pork chop is definitely an American standard. The chops are probably best cooked on a ridged griddle, but a heavy cast-iron skillet will do a fine job.

¼ cup fresh thyme leaves
1 teaspoon salt
1 teaspoon black pepper, freshly ground
1 clove garlic, peeled
Zest and juice of 1 lemon
1 tablespoon hazelnut oil
4 two-rib pork chops

In a food processor, add the thyme and salt and lightly pulse. Add the garlic and pepper and lightly pulse again. Stir in the lemon juice and zest and oil and pulse until well mixed. Rub the chops with the mixture and let them marinate for about 15 minutes.

Preheat the griddle over medium-high heat until it is very hot. Place the chops on the hot griddle and step back; there could be a lot of smoke. You want the chops to be charred and nicely golden. If they start to brown too much, turn down the heat. Cook for about 7 minutes on each side. Don't overcook the chops, or the meat will become dry. Take the chops off the griddle, and let them sit for about 3 minutes before serving them.

Good for A, B, and C dieters.

Braised Pork Roast with Olives

SERVES 6.

Janet W. sent this recipe to me from Larchmont, New York. She wanted to combine her love of olives with a healthy way of preparing meat. Combined, she and members of her family have lost more than 200 pounds. She loves this meal on a cold, snowy day.

1 tablespoon macadamia nut oil
1 3½-pound rack of pork, 6 ribs, boned, and tied to
   the rack of bones
5 cloves garlic, minced
½ cup red onion, chopped
3 bay leaves
½ cup red wine vinegar
½ cup cooking red wine
1 cup chicken stock
Salt
White pepper, freshly ground
¼ cup kalamata olives, sliced
1 tablespoon flat-leaf parsley, chopped
1 tablespoon thyme, chopped

Heat the oil in a large Dutch oven over medium-high heat. Allow the oil to almost reach its smoke point, then add the pork, and sear it on all sides until lightly browned, about 20 minutes. Don't be afraid of this step. Remove the meat. Add the garlic and onions and sauté until soft but not brown. Add the bay leaves, then deglaze the pan with the vinegar. Add the red wine and the chicken stock. Season the pork with salt and pepper and return it to the pot.

Allow the pork to cook over a low heat for about 45 minutes, basting occasionally. Discard the bay leaves. Remove the meat to a platter and let it rest for 20 minutes. Reheat the sauce and add the olives, parsley, and thyme.

Separate the ribs onto a different plate, spoon the sauce over each rib, and serve.

Good for A, B, and C dieters.

Pork Tenderloin with Cream Sauce

SERVES 6.

When I visited my friend Heidi, who lives in Dallas, she served this dish to me for dinner. Besides being delicious, it is one of the simplest preparations of an impressive main course I can imagine.

Macadamia nut oil
3 or 4 shallots, diced
Salt
Black pepper, freshly ground
4 pounds pork tenderloin, rolled and tied
4 cups organic chicken broth
1 pint organic half-and-half

Heat some macadamia nut oil in a roasting pot. Add the shallots and sauté until transparent. Coat the pork loin with salt and pepper and add it to the pot. Sear the pork on all sides. Pour the chicken broth and half-and-half over the pork. Turn down the heat to a simmer and cover the pot. Slowly simmer for 2 hours, turning the pork every so often and stirring gravy. Remove the pork from the pot to let it rest and tightly cover it with aluminum foil. Return the pot to the heat and cook the gravy until it reduces and thickens. Slice the pork into slices three-quarters of an inch thick and return the pork to the pot to coat with the gravy before serving.

Good for A, B, and C dieters.

Broiled Veal Chops with Sage and Rosemary

SERVES 4.

Jan R. from Denmark sent me this recipe. It's one of his family's favorites, especially during the cold fall and winter evenings that start in October in his native country. He lost 45 pounds, his wife lost 30, and even his teenager dropped a few pounds just by learning to eat more healthy.

4 10-ounce veal chops, bone in
2 garlic cloves, peeled and halved
Salt
Red pepper, freshly ground
1 tablespoon macadamia nut oil
1 large chipotle chili packed in adobo sauce (I would use a
    dried or fresh chipotle pepper), minced
1½ teaspoons of the adobo sauce from the can of chilis (or make
    your own adobo sauce, as described in the recipe)
2 teaspoons lo-han (Since this is not for a glaze, stevia,
    Splenda, or even saccharin would also do the trick.)
2 teaspoons fresh sage, chopped
2 teaspoons fresh rosemary, chopped

To make your own adobo sauce, take the chipotle pepper, either fresh (preferred) or dried (the latter would have to be soaked in water), and chop it well; add 1 stewed tomato and ½ teaspoon of vinegar, and marinate for as long as you need to. This sauce can be made a long time in advance and enough can be made to save for future recipes.

Vigorously rub the veal chops with the cut side of the garlic cloves to allow the garlic's oil to be released. Season the chops with salt and pepper. In a small bowl, mix the macadamia nut oil, chipotle chili, adobo sauce, and lo-han. Pour the mixture over the chops and rub each side to get a good coating. Let them marinate for at least 30 minutes and up to 24 hours in the refrigerator to allow the heat to settle in.

When you're ready to cook the chops, preheat the oven to broil. Set the chops on a cookie sheet or broiler pan and place under the flame for about 5 minutes on each side for medium rare—longer for well done. Allow to rest for 5 minutes, sprinkle with the chopped herbs, and serve.

Good for A, B, and C dieters.

Spicy Buffalo Meatballs in Mushroom Cream Sauce

SERVES 2.

Just when you thought that meatballs of any sort would be a boring variation on a hamburger—surprise! This dish makes a great main course that will excite your palate.

1 pound ground organic buffalo
1 egg
¼ cup grated Parmesan cheese
½ teaspoon salt
¼ cup chopped Italian parsley
2 tablespoons chopped roasted red pepper
1 jalapeño pepper, seeded and diced
Macadamia nut oil
1 cup button mushrooms, sliced
½ pint organic heavy cream
Salt
Black pepper, freshly ground
3 big handfuls of baby spinach

In a large bowl, mix together the buffalo, egg, cheese, salt, parsley, and red and jalapeño peppers. You may adjust the amount of jalapeño depending on your individual taste. Form meatballs about the size of golf balls. Place them in a cast-iron skillet with some macadamia nut oil. Sauté and turn as needed until the meatballs are cooked through.

While the meatballs are cooking, sauté the mushrooms in a saucepan with some macadamia nut oil until they are cooked down. Place the mushrooms into a blender with the cream and blend until a sauce forms. Salt and pepper the sauce to taste.

On a serving plate, form a bed out of the baby spinach. Top the spinach with the meatballs. Pour the cream sauce over the meatballs and serve. The heat from the buffalo meatballs and mushroom sauce will wilt the spinach.

Good for A, B, and C dieters.

Vegetarian Moussaka

SERVES 6.

Even vegetarians can eat in a healthier way by restricting their intake of simple carbohydrates and sugars. This recipe was sent to me by dear friends from Boston who loved the Hamptons Diet and who have been vegetarians since college. For strict vegans, you can omit the egg and the cheese.

1 medium eggplant, peeled
Sea salt
4 small carrots, quartered
2 large stalks celery, quartered
1 medium yellow onion, quartered
¼ cup macadamia nut oil
¼ cup pine nuts
3 large garlic cloves, minced
2 portobello mushrooms, diced
1 teaspoon oregano, minced
1 teaspoon cinnamon
½ teaspoon ground nutmeg
2 cups tomato sauce, sugar-free
¼ cup flat-leaf parsley, minced
1½ cups ricotta cheese
1 egg yolk
1 cup Parmesan cheese, grated

Preheat the oven to 350°F. Slice the eggplant into ¼-inch slices, salt both sides, and place on paper towels.

Put the carrots, celery, and onions into a food processor and chop them. Heat 2 tablespoons of macadamia nut oil in a skillet over medium-high heat. Add the mixture from the food processor and sauté until the onions turn golden. Add the pine nuts, garlic, mushrooms, oregano, cinnamon, nutmeg, tomato sauce, and parsley. Turn down the heat and simmer.

Toss the eggplant with the remaining oil. Arrange the eggplant on a cookie sheet so the slices don't overlap. Bake for 20 minutes.

Put the ricotta in a saucepan over low heat. Whisk in the egg yolk and ½ cup of Parmesan cheese. Beat well. Remove from the heat.

Lightly grease a glass soufflé dish. Place a layer of eggplant on the bottom and spoon the tomato sauce mixture over it. Make two more layers of eggplant and sauce. Top these layers with the ricotta mixture. Sprinkle the dish with the remaining ½ cup of Parmesan cheese.

Bake it at 350°F for 40 minutes (or until the cheese is golden brown).

Moussaka, Nonvegetarian Variation

Add 1 pound of ground lamb while the onions are sautéing. Omit 1 tablespoon of oil and the celery and carrots.

Good for B and C dieters.

Portobello Steak

SERVES 4 AS A MAIN COURSE. SERVES 8 AS A SIDE DISH.

Here is another vegetarian entrée suggestion. It also makes a great side dish for those of us who like to eat meat. Again, for the strict vegan, omit the cheese and the egg. This recipe was sent to me by Edna W. from Waco, Texas. Although she has lived on a working ranch most of her life, she refuses to eat the animals, and since she loves the Hamptons Diet so much, she wanted to share something that to her tastes better than a juicy steak.

4 large portobello mushrooms with stems
3 tablespoons macadamia nut oil
1 pound fresh spinach, chopped
1 large onion, chopped
2 tablespoons garlic, chopped
½ cup pine nuts
2 eggs
½ cup Parmesan cheese
½ cup fresh flat-leaf parsley, chopped
¼ cup fresh chervil, chopped
½ teaspoon sea salt
½ teaspoon white pepper
3 drops of hot pepper sauce (optional)
1 cup mozzarella cheese, shredded

Preheat the oven to 375°F.

Remove the stems from the mushrooms. Cut off the ends of the stems. Wash and dry the stems, then chop and set aside. Place the caps in a baking dish with the top sides down.

Heat the oil over medium heat in a skillet. Sauté the stems, spinach, onion, garlic, and nuts in the oil until the nuts are lightly golden. Combine the eggs, Parmesan, parsley, and chervil, and add the salt, pepper, and hot sauce. Pour the mixture over the sautéed vegetables and mix well. Spoon a quarter of the mixture onto each mushroom cap. Sprinkle with grated mozzarella.

Bake for 30 to 45 minutes or until browned.

Good for B and C dieters. Good for A dieters if used as a side dish.

Grilled Vegetables

A book about the Hamptons wouldn't be complete without a section on grilling. I especially love to grill vegetables, but up until this year, I was terrible at it. For some reason, the vegetables always fell through the cracks onto the flames. This year, I bought a vegetable grill gadget that keeps them in between two pieces of metal so that they don't fall through.

Although grilling is primarily considered a summer activity, I recommend that you do it in the winter as well. The food is hearty and can thoroughly warm you up on cold winter evenings. Think how surprised your guests will be to be served a grilled dinner in the dead of winter.

Grilling is an easy way to make a great-tasting and healthy meal. Grilled meals can be prepared and cooked quickly, and they are filled with protein and delicious vegetables. Wood can also be used in a gas grill, if you buy a special attachment for the grill.

One of Jeff's tricks to guarantee a great savory grilled flavor is throwing on some wood chips when the coals are red. Once the flames have died down, the fire is ready for both cooking and the addition of your choice of wood chips. The best woods to use are maple, cherry, mesquite, apple, or pear. Never use pine or eucalyptus; they are too resinous and make a complete mess without adding much flavor.

Chef Jeff recommends that in the summertime, when you're grilling up burgers or ribs, you might as well throw on some fresh vegetables. The following vegetables are his favorites. I recommend that you always choose vegetables according to what is fresh, local, and seasonal—this will make any meal extra healthy.

The great thing about grilled vegetables is that they can be served hot or at room temperature. They can also be cooked ahead of time and arranged on a large serving plate before your guests arrive. I like to cook things that I can mess up when no one else is in my kitchen, and I'm not sipping my other favorite clear liquid—vodka.

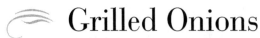

Grilled Onions

SERVES 4.

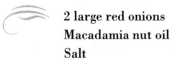

2 large red onions
Macadamia nut oil
Salt

Peel the onions, and slice them about a third of an inch thick. Lightly brush the onions with oil and add a sprinkle of salt. Grill for about 6 minutes on each side or until they darken around the edges and the rings start to separate. Beware, they may drop through to the coals if you don't have a vegetable grill accessory. You may use fewer onions if you are grilling a mélange of vegetables, which is something I always recommend—the more colorful the better. Not only will they look better plated, but they will be at their healthiest this way.

Good for A, B, and C dieters.

Grilled Fennel

SERVES 4.

Don't be afraid of this vegetable. It looks a little odd but is a taste sensation. Treat it like a type of onion. Grilled fennel wedges look great and have a slight licorice flavor. They are loaded with vitamins and minerals, too.

2 medium fennel bulbs
Macadamia nut oil

Cut off the stems of the fennel bulb if they are still attached and cut off the bulb about a half inch from the bottom. Cut the bulb down the middle, length-wise in half, then cut the halves into 3 or 4 wedges. Toss with macadamia nut oil and grill for 10 to 12 minutes on each side, until light brown.

Good for A, B, and C dieters.

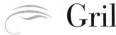

Grilled Eggplant

SERVES 4.

Eggplant is quick and easy to grill. Jeff likes to sprinkle eggplant with fresh herbs from the garden, and I couldn't agree more. Cooking Hamptons Diet style means making each meal its healthiest. Why not add vegetables in any way you can?

1½ pounds eggplant
Macadamia nut oil
Salt
Black pepper, freshly ground

Fresh herbs, chopped (whatever is seasonal but, certainly, mint, rosemary, thyme, or basil will be exceptional with this dish)

   Slice the eggplant crosswise into rounds. Jeff tells us not to bother peeling the eggplant when we grill it. Brush each slice with a little macadamia nut oil and add salt, pepper, and fresh herbs if you like. Grill the slices for about 7 minutes on each side or until well browned.

Good for A, B, and C dieters.

Grilled Portobello Mushrooms

Grill spillage alert for this one! I have never to this day successfully grilled a portobello mushroom without the use of a grill gadget. So if you try this without the aid of that little parachute, don't blame me if it falls into the fire.

4 large portobello mushrooms
3 tablespoons macadamia nut oil
1 tablespoon fresh thyme, chopped
Salt
Black pepper, freshly ground

Pull the stems off the mushroom caps. In a small bowl, combine the macadamia nut oil, thyme, salt, and pepper with a wire whisk. Brush the mushrooms on each side with this mixture. Set the mixture aside; you will need it to brush each mushroom several times during the grilling process. Place the mushrooms about 7 inches from the coals and grill for about 10 to 12 minutes or until they start to release liquid and are slightly soft to the touch.

Good for A, B, and C dieters.

Grilled Asparagus

SERVES 4.

Asparagus is very easy to grill, but remember my caveat about vegetables that fall into the coals. The easiest way to know the correct place to trim the asparagus is to let the stalk guide you. Hold each end of an asparagus spear with one hand and gently bend it. The stalk will bend exactly where it needs to be trimmed.

1 pound asparagus spears, white or green, depending on
    the season
½ cup macadamia nut oil
Salt

Trim the ends off the asparagus as described previously. In a separate bowl, mix the oil and salt together with a wire whisk. Toss the asparagus spears in the oil mixture and then grill for about 8 to 10 minutes or until heated through and slightly brown. Serve them.

Good for A, B, and C dieters.

Grilled Wild King Salmon

SERVES 4–6.

Jeff lived in Anchorage, Alaska, for a year and said he has never eaten as much delicious salmon in his life as he ate there. One evening he and his friends were sitting on his back deck, grilling some king salmon and watching the sun go down, when a friend asked what time it was. To his amazement, it was 11:30 P.M. and the sun was just reaching the horizon. They enjoyed some spectacular grilled king salmon around midnight, sitting on that back deck.

If you turn to the resource section, you can find a great source for this type of salmon. It is seasonal and somewhat difficult to find on the East Coast. My source can send it to you frozen, and it is out-of-this-world delicious.

4–7 fillets king salmon
Salt
White pepper, freshly ground
Macadamia nut oil

Take the salmon out of the refrigerator at least 30 minutes before grilling it. If using frozen fillets, thaw them before starting this recipe.

Heat the grill for 10 to 15 minutes before using it if it's electric or gas. If using charcoal, make sure the charcoals are gray and pink, with no black spots or flames, and be sure to have the grate about 7 inches above the coals. This will probably be about 60 minutes after you first ignite the flames. Regardless of the type of fire, clean the grill with a wire brush and then wipe it with a pre-oiled cloth to prevent the fish from sticking to it.

Season the fish with salt and pepper. Rub it with oil and place the fish, skin-side down, on the grill. Grill until medium rare, about 5 minutes on each side. This salmon can be served with a grilled vegetable, such as asparagus. The Malaga Vinaigrette found in the next chapter would be a nice sauce for this fish.

Good for A, B, and C dieters.

Grilled Halibut with Teriyaki

SERVES 4.

Halibut is one of my favorite fish. It has a delicate buttery flavor and can be roasted to perfection. It's a perfect dish to serve to guests because the fish will take on the flavor of the sauce it's served with, and you don't have to worry about offending guests whose palate is less developed than yours and who like only nonfishy fish. This is a definite nonfishy fish and is a great one to try with the kids to see whether they'll eat it.

Halibut can also be ordered from the company I mention in the resource section. It sends some of the best wild halibut I have ever eaten directly to your door. Because the fish is from Alaska, there is no need to worry as much about the mercury or the PCB levels found in it.

4 8-ounce halibut steaks

Take the halibut out of the refrigerator at least 30 minutes before grilling it. Heat the grill for 10 to 15 minutes before using it if it's electric or gas. If you're using charcoal, make sure the charcoals are gray and pink, with no black spots or flames, and be sure to have the grate about 7 inches above the coals. Clean the grill with a wire brush and then wipe it with a pre-oiled cloth to prevent the fish from sticking to it.

Make the marinade. Do not refrigerate unless you're making it ahead of time. Add the halibut to the marinade and let sit for about 30 minutes before grilling it. Grill for about 7 minutes on each side.

Fish Marinade
MAKES ¾ CUP.

½ cup light soy sauce
3 tablespoons mirin (Japanese rice wine)
6 drops Tabasco sauce (optional)

In a small saucepan, heat the soy sauce, mirin, and Tabasco (if you're using it), and reduce the liquid by half. Pour the marinade into a medium-size glass bowl and cool it to room temperature.

Good for A, B, and C dieters.

Grilled Hanger Steak

SERVES 4.

This cut of meat is one of Jeff's favorites to throw on the grill. It is relatively inexpensive and very tender, and it has a deep rich flavor. Because it's so flavorful, he likes to season it only with salt and pepper. This is a cut of meat that you may need to ask a butcher about. You most likely won't be able to find this cut in the meat department of a supermarket, but you may be able to ask the butcher to get some before it's ground into hamburger meat.

4 6-ounce hanger steaks
Salt
Black pepper, freshly ground
Macadamia nut oil

Season the steak with salt and pepper about 4 hours before you're going to grill it or even the night before. Then refrigerate, covered, until 30 minutes before grilling. Press the meat dry between paper towels and rub it with the oil.

The cooking time for this dish can vary greatly, depending on how thick your steaks are, the desired degree of doneness, how hot the grill is, and so on. Prepare the grill as described previously. Place the meat on the grill. For medium rare, grill for about 8 minutes on each side. Because of the many variables, this is just a suggestion; make sure the steak is nicely colored from the grill on the outside before removing it from the heat. When it's done, take it off the grill and let it sit for a few minutes before slicing it.

Slice it straight across the grain. Cutting strategically across the grain minimizes the "chewiness" problem and allows your steak to be its most tender. When cutting steak this way, you will get a collection of oval and oblong slices. Jeff likes to serve this steak with grilled portobello mushrooms and a light mixed green salad. This dinner can be enjoyed any time of year.

Good for A, B, and C dieters.

Grilled Sausages

SERVES 4.

Today in the marketplace there are so many different kinds of sausage. Pick out whatever sausage you or your family enjoy; there is certainly one to suit any palate. Turkey apple, chicken fennel, pork with Asian spices, and so on.

Chef Jeff tells us, "Pick out a nice fat one, and stoke up the barbie." One little trick to cooking sausage on the grill is to poke about 10 holes in the sausage with a toothpick to prevent its cracking or exploding.

6 sausages of your choice

Heat up the grill, as described previously, and throw on the sausages. Flip over the sausages every 3 minutes or so until cooked all the way through.

Any grilled sausage would go well with grilled onions and perhaps a grilled fruit, such as cantaloupe, peach, or apple. I also serve these sausages over a seasonal salad for a nice, light, yet very filling, lunch.

Good for A, B, and C dieters.

Braised Brussels Sprouts with Bacon and Sour Cream

SERVES 4.

This dish is a favorite of my friend Tom's. It soon became a favorite of mine as well.

8 ounces organic bacon
2 shallots, diced
2 pounds Brussels sprouts, bottoms removed
½ cup organic chicken broth
8 ounces organic sour cream
2 tablespoons white horseradish
¼ cup Parmesan cheese, freshly grated
Salt and pepper to taste

Put the bacon in a heated cast-iron skillet. When the bacon is crispy, remove it from the skillet and set it aside on a paper towel to drain. Discard half of the bacon fat from the skillet. Add the shallots to the skillet and sauté until they are transparent. Add the Brussels sprouts and sauté until they begin to braise. Pour in the chicken broth and cook, covered, for 10 to 15 minutes. Remove the cover and continue to braise the sprouts until they are cooked through and have a beautiful patina. Crumble the bacon. Mix the sour cream, horseradish, Parmesan cheese, and crumbled bacon into the skillet. Add salt and pepper to taste and serve.

Good for A, B, and C dieters.

⤶ 6 ⤷

Hamptons Diet
Side Dishes and Salads

Y ou can create so many wonderful side dishes as part of a healthy
eating lifestyle. In this section, I encourage you to mix and match
these recipes. Often, one vegetable can be easily exchanged for another.
You will never again be able to use boredom as an excuse for going off your
diet. The side dishes presented here are delicious, and I often make a meal
of several of them. Jeff learned many of these recipes in Spain and was
influenced by the tapas culture. For me, I always remember going to dinners and wanting three or four sides instead of a meal. The best thing about
sides is that they can be reheated over and over again, and they usually get
better each time they are reheated.

There are many side-dish salads. Between the salads in this chapter and
the ones in the lunch chapter, you should be able to master the art of salad
making. Don't be afraid to experiment. You can serve these salads any time

of the day. One of the joys of cooking is that you can do things however you like.

The hardest thing for me is to get a salad to look pretty. When you go to restaurants, the salads come out looking so perfect and delicious. Mine reach the table tasting great but lacking in the aesthetic department. My guests never seem to complain, though, so I must be doing something right—or maybe they are just polite!

Winter Waldorf Salad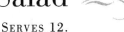

SERVES 12.

This was sent to me by Sarah B. She loves this salad so much that, as a special treat, she serves it in martini glasses when she entertains. Also, she tends to change up the apple varieties in it dish, depending on what's available at the farm stand that day. It's a great salad for cold fall or winter nights.

¾ cup maconnaise (see recipe, page 73)

¾ cup sour cream or crème fraîche

1½ tablespoons lime juice

¾ teaspoon ginger, freshly grated

3 large Granny Smith apples, chopped

3 large red apples, chopped (Red Delicious—although I don't like these types of apples—are the most common and are found in most supermarkets)

3 large yellow apples, chopped (Golden Delicious)

½ cup celery, diced

1½ cups walnuts, toasted, chopped

In a large bowl, whisk together the first four ingredients. Then add the rest of the ingredients and refrigerate the salad for about 1 hour or until ready to serve. Because of the lime juice, the apples will not turn brown.

Good for B and C dieters.

Picadilla (Creamy Almond Salad Dressing)

MAKES 1¼ CUPS.

This dressing hails from Valencia in the southern part of Spain and is Jeff's interpretation of the classic. Almond, olive, and lemon trees grow abundantly throughout that region, and the fruits of these three trees make up this wonderful dressing, which can be used with a salad or poached fish.

½ cup blanched almonds
4 cloves garlic, minced
½ teaspoon salt
4 teaspoons sherry vinegar
4 teaspoons lemon juice, freshly squeezed
Black pepper, freshly ground
1 cup extra-virgin olive oil (or macadamia nut oil,
    to make this even healthier)

Grind the almonds with the garlic in a food processor or blender. Add the salt, vinegar, lemon juice, and pepper. Gradually pour in the oil until the dressing is creamy and smooth.

Good for A, B, and C dieters.

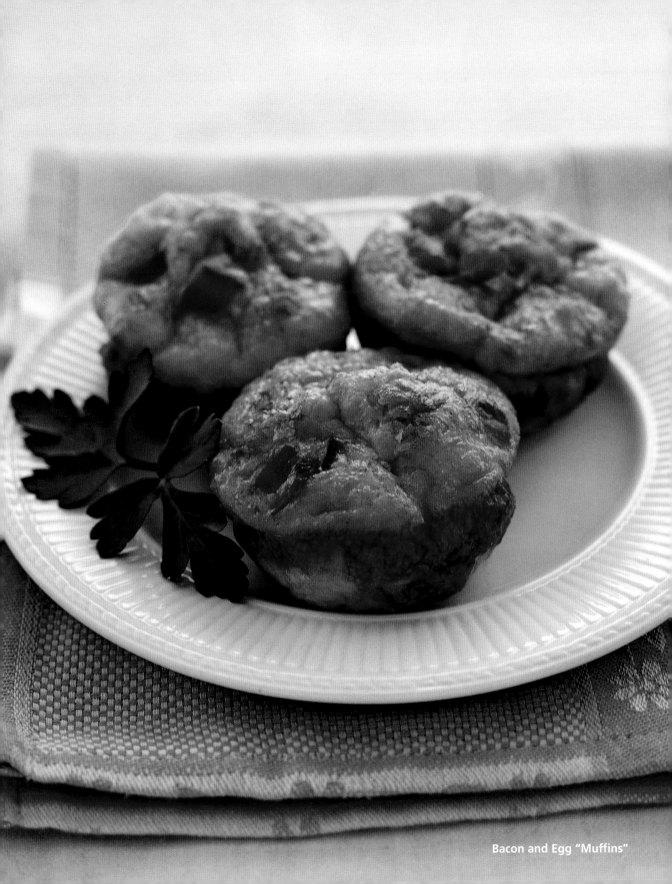

Bacon and Egg "Muffins"

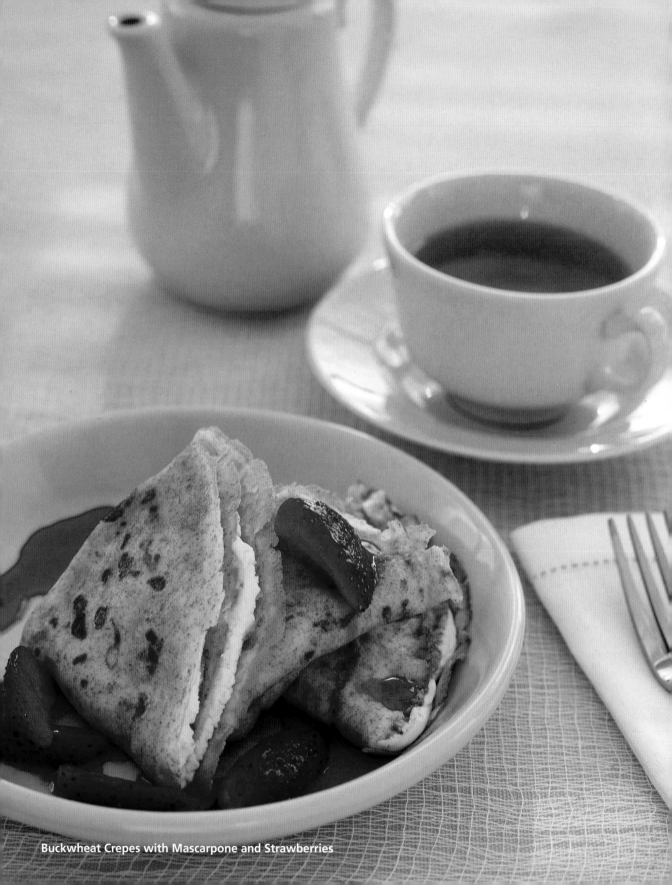

Buckwheat Crepes with Mascarpone and Strawberries

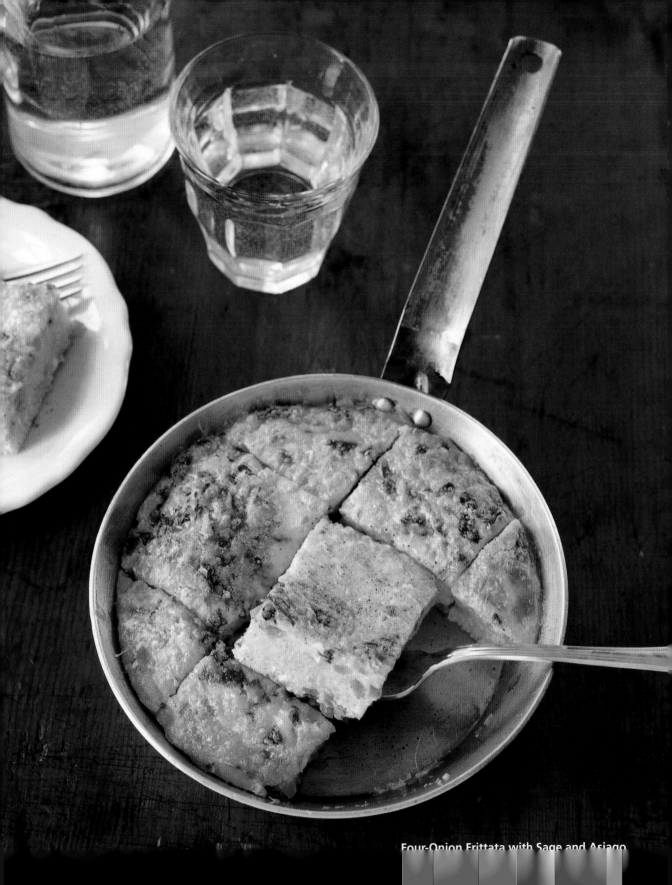

Four-Onion Frittata with Sage and Asiago

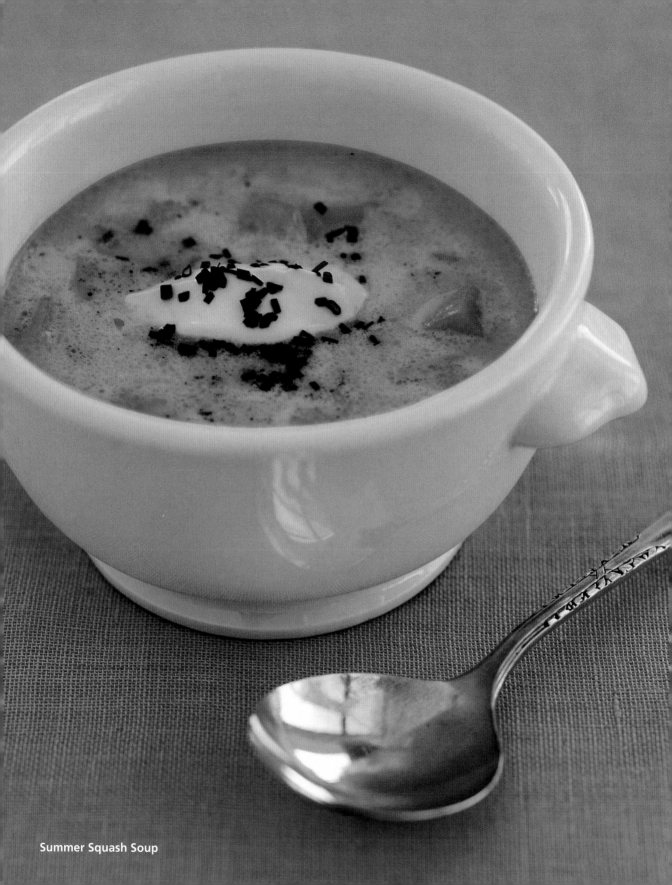

Summer Squash Soup

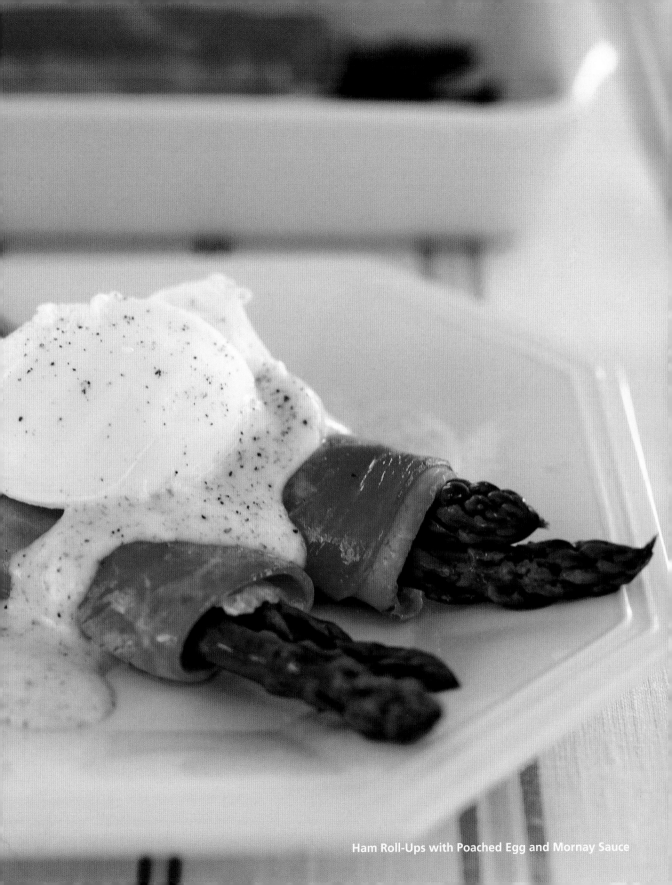

Ham Roll-Ups with Poached Egg and Mornay Sauce

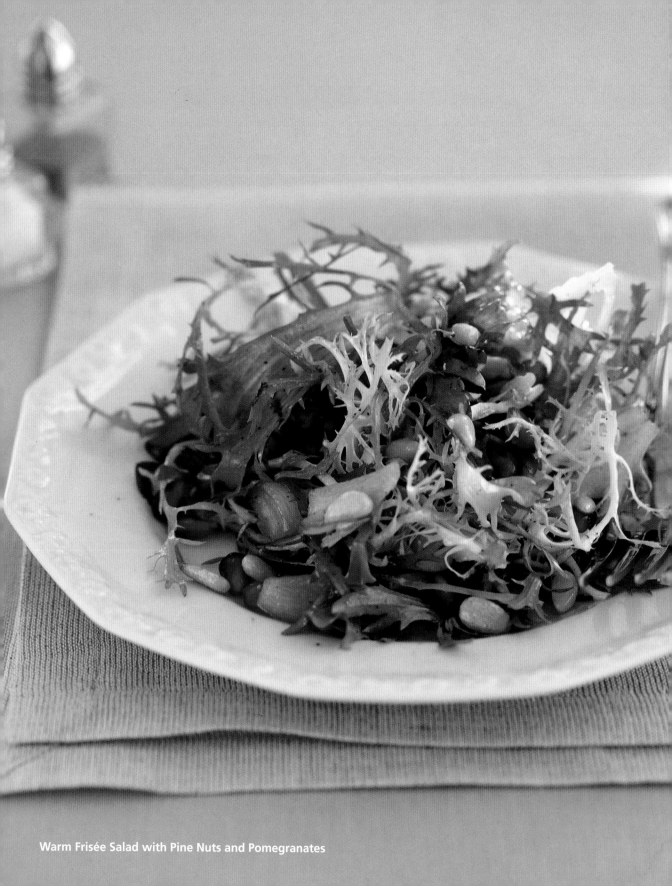

Warm Frisée Salad with Pine Nuts and Pomegranates

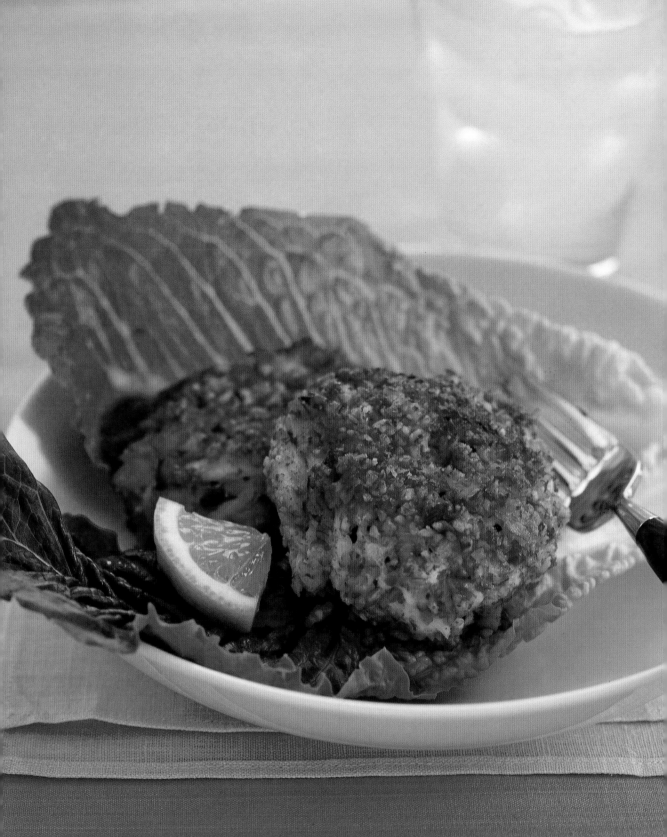

Southampton Crab Cakes

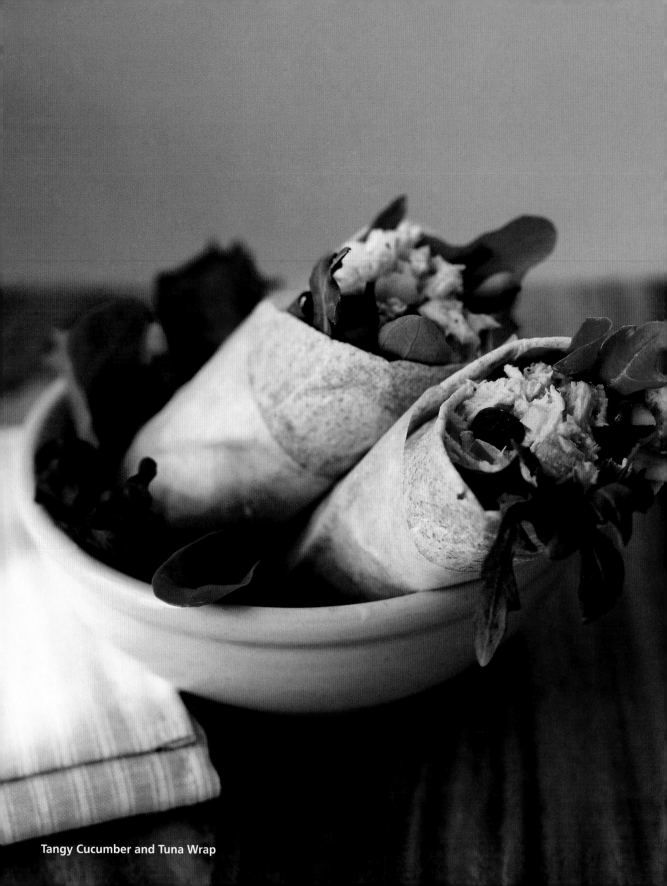

Tangy Cucumber and Tuna Wrap

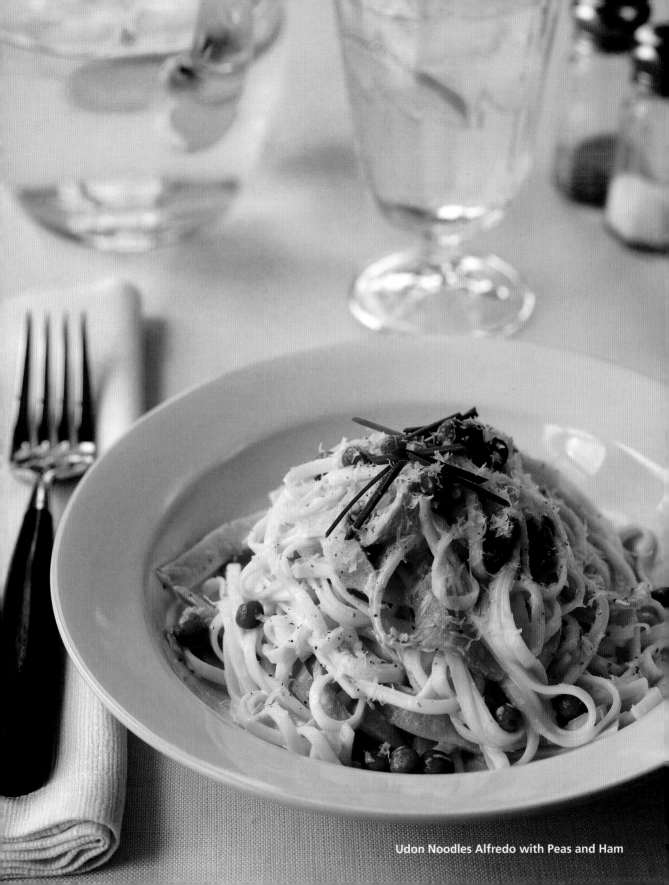
Udon Noodles Alfredo with Peas and Ham

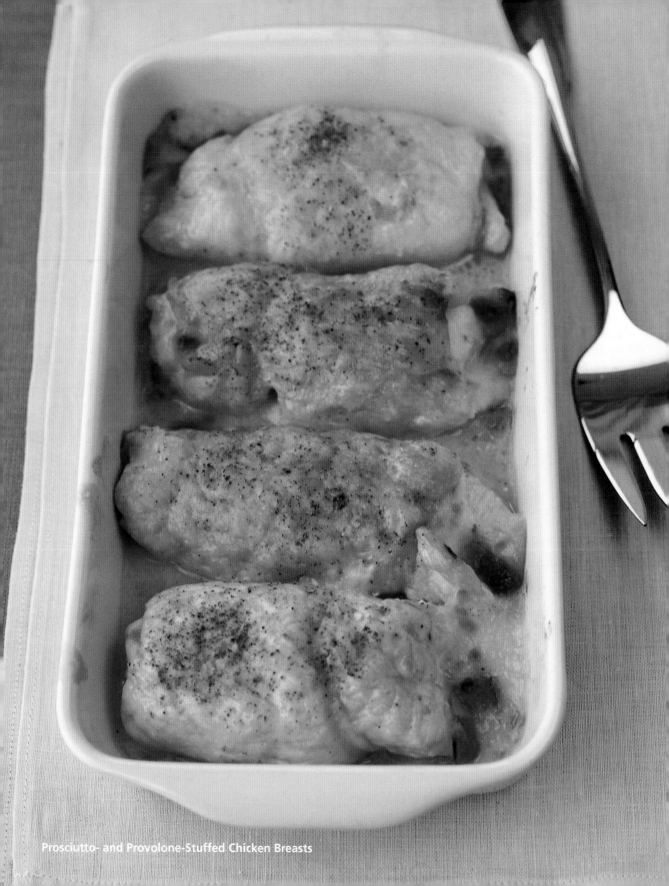

Prosciutto- and Provolone-Stuffed Chicken Breasts

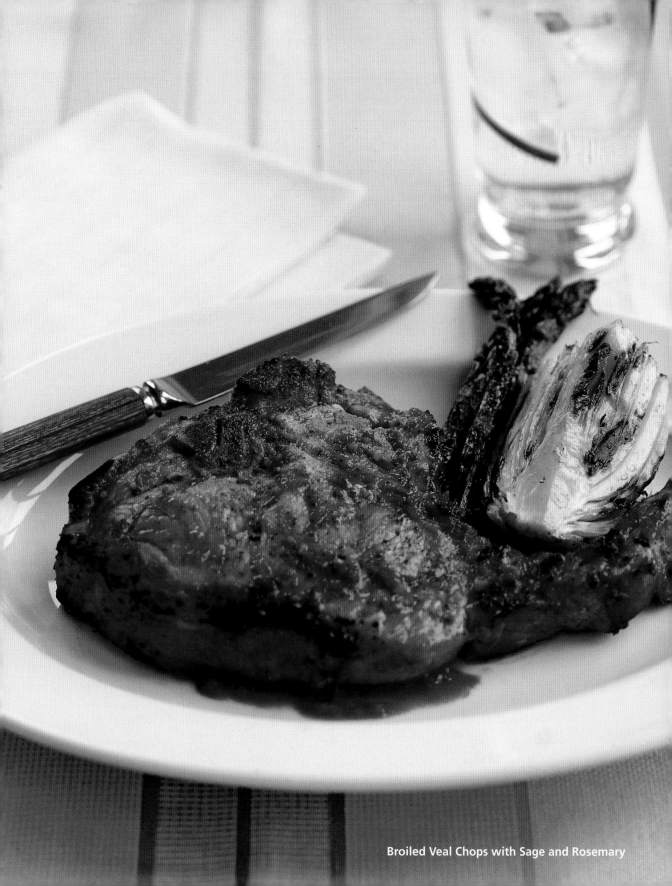

Broiled Veal Chops with Sage and Rosemary

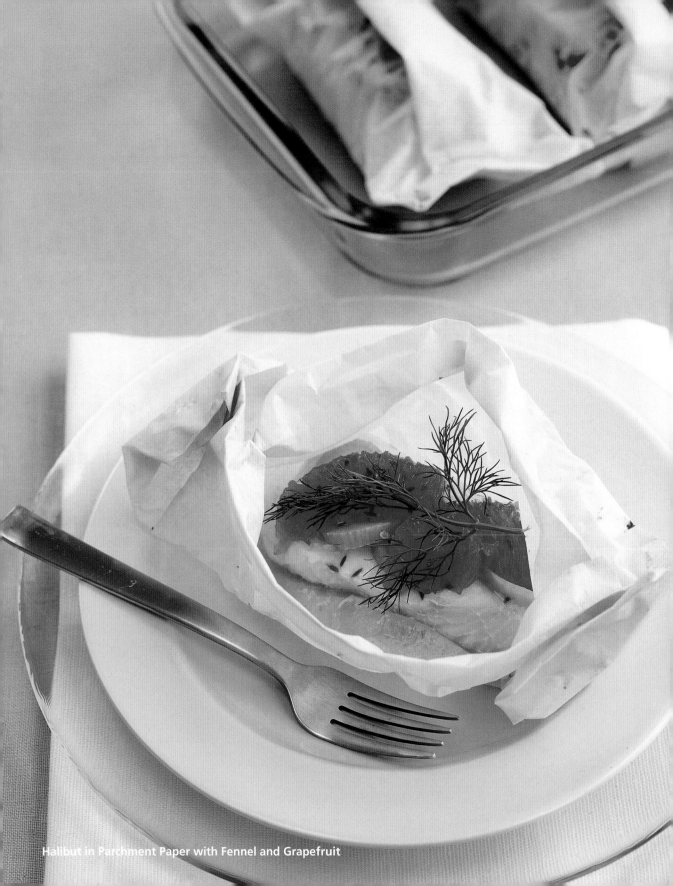

Halibut in Parchment Paper with Fennel and Grapefruit

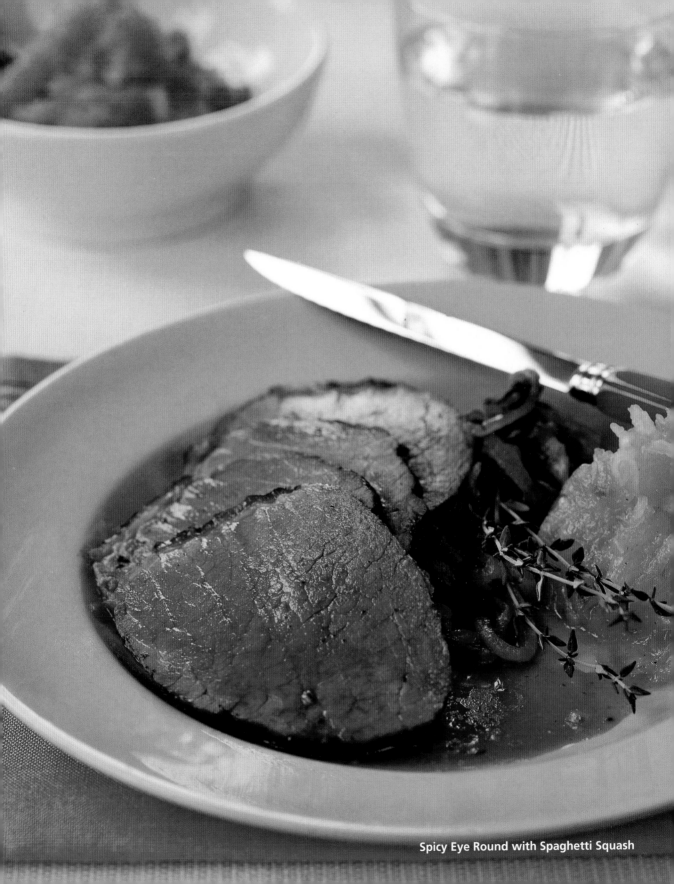

Spicy Eye Round with Spaghetti Squash

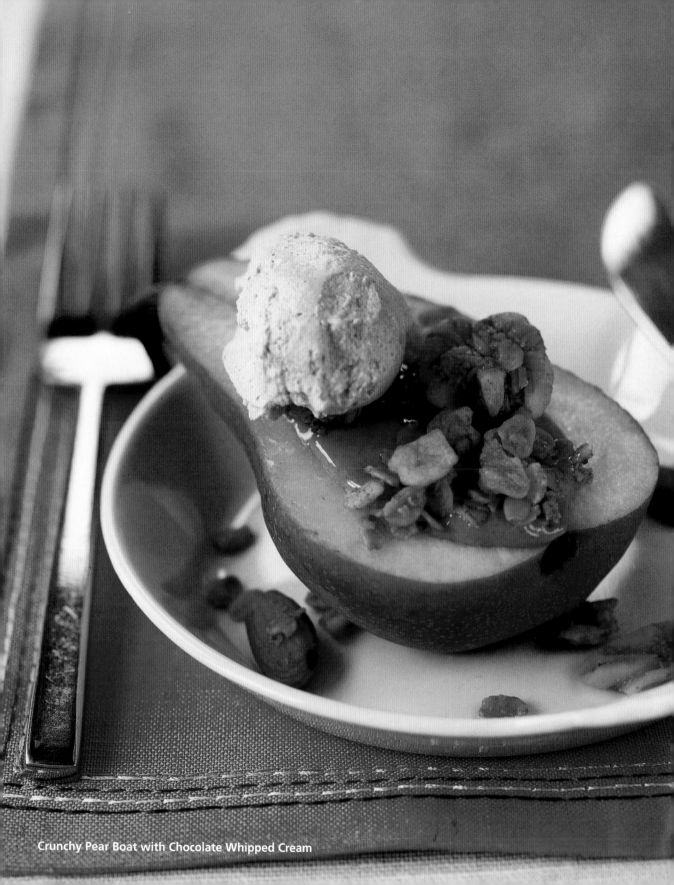

Crunchy Pear Boat with Chocolate Whipped Cream

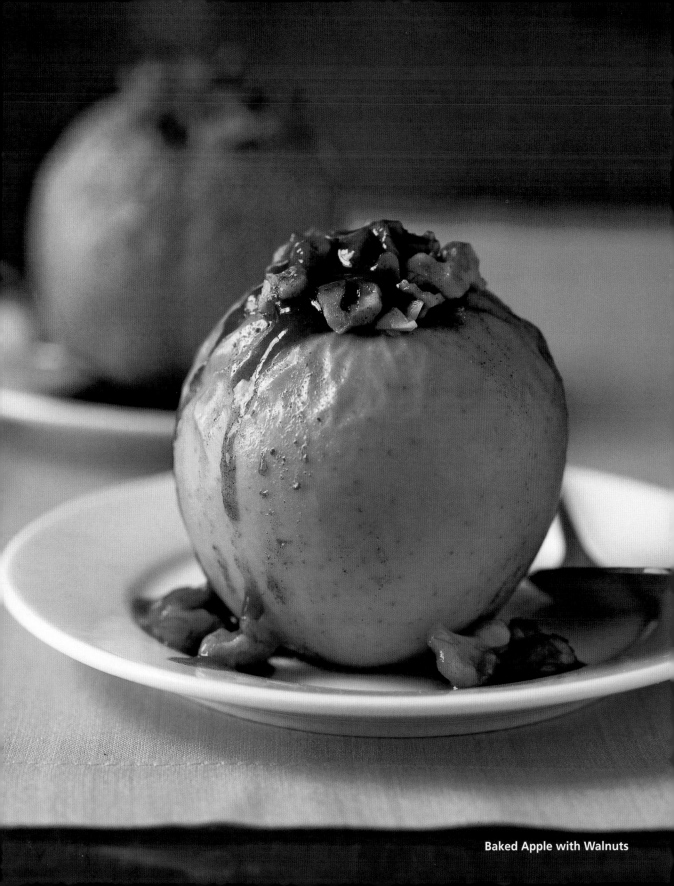

Baked Apple with Walnuts

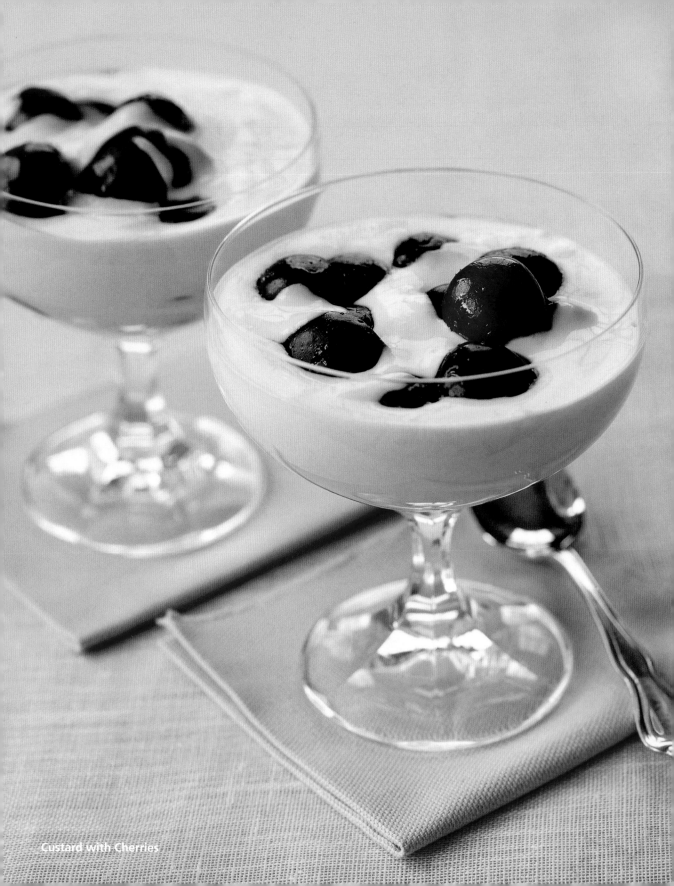

Custard with Cherries

Ensalada Mixta

SERVES 4.

This simple salad is found all over Spain. The key ingredients are onion, tomato, lettuce, and tuna. You can add ingredients or take some away as you wish. Master this salad, and you can always make a quick lunch or dinner side dish.

2 tablespoons red wine vinegar
¼ cup macadamia nut oil
Salt
Black pepper, freshly ground
1 head romaine lettuce, torn into pieces and rinsed
2 ripe tomatoes, cut in eighths (optional)
¼ red onion, thinly sliced
6 spears white asparagus
12 small green Spanish olives
7-ounce can albacore tuna in water, drained

In a small bowl blend the vinegar, oil, salt, and pepper. In a salad bowl, gently mix together the lettuce, optional tomato, onion, asparagus, olives, and tuna. Pour the vinaigrette onto the salad and toss. Divide the salad among four individual salad plates or serve it in a big bowl and let people help themselves.

Good for A, B, and C dieters.

Mixed Salad with Hazelnuts and Goat Cheese

SERVES 4.

Jeff prefers to serve this salad before duck, pheasant, or lamb. Those dishes are a little hard for me to make, except for maybe lamb. I guess that's why he's the chef and I'm the physician. In any case, this is a nice fall salad.

½ cup hazelnuts
¼ cup extra-virgin olive oil
1 tablespoon macadamia nut oil
1 tablespoon champagne vinegar
Salt
6 ounces mesclun greens, washed and dried
4 ounces goat cheese, thinly sliced

Preheat the oven to 350°F.

Spread the hazelnuts on a baking sheet and roast until the skins darken, about 10 minutes. While they're still hot, rub the hazelnuts in a clean dish towel to remove the skins. Chop coarsely.

In a medium bowl add the oils, vinegar, and salt, and beat well with a whisk. In another large bowl add the lettuce, half of the hazelnuts, and the oil and vinegar mixture. Mix well. Plate the salad on a serving platter and top with the remaining hazelnuts and the goat cheese.

Good for A, B, and C dieters.

Fennel and Grapefruit Salad

In Italy, fennel is greatly appreciated, and the fronds of wild fennel are often used to flavor dishes. Fennel tastes a lot like licorice and is a strong, yet subtle, flavor. I first learned of fennel's medicinal qualities while I was in Italy during medical school. Fennel has digestive enzymes in the bulb and is often served as either an appetizer or after the main meal simply to cleanse the palate. This makes it an extremely healthy component to any diet, but it is not yet all that popular in the United States.

This simple salad pairs raw fennel with grapefruit, dressed with extra-virgin olive oil, salt, and pepper. Jeff used to make this salad at wedding parties in Italy, and everyone always loved it.

1 grapefruit
2 fennel bulbs, halved and thinly sliced
3 tablespoons extra-virgin olive oil
Coarse sea salt
White pepper, freshly ground

Slice both ends off the grapefruit, cutting just deeply enough to expose the flesh. Setting the fruit on one cut end, use a paring knife to carve away the skin and pith in a series of smooth, arcing strokes from top to bottom, rotating the fruit with each stroke as you work your way around the grapefruit. Then cut out each segment, working over a bowl to catch the juice. In a large bowl, combine the grapefruit segments, retained grapefruit juice, sliced fennel, olive oil, salt, and pepper. Toss well, divide into four plates, and serve. In Italy, this salad is served on a large plate at the end of the meal for the diners to pick through—a more rustic presentation but more authentic and equally delicious.

Good for A, B, and C dieters.

Heirloom Tomato, Mozzarella, and Basil Salad

SERVES 3.

This is the Hamptons version of the famous Caprese salad from Capri. At Alison restaurant, Jeff makes this salad from local heirloom tomatoes, buffalo mozzarella from Cavaniola's (the local cheese shop), and freshly picked basil from the restaurant's herb garden. Now, that spells Hamptons Diet all the way—fresh, local, and seasonal. This makes a perfect midsummer lunch dish and a great summer dinner salad to serve at a barbecue. It's a simple salad to master and one that everyone loves.

3 large tomatoes, different-colored
1 fresh mozzarella ball, medium-sized
9 basil leaves, medium-sized
2 tablespoons balsamic vinegar
6 tablespoons macadamia nut oil
Salt
Black pepper, freshly ground

Slice each tomato so that you get 3 slices from each, 9 altogether. Slice the mozzarella into 9 thin slices. Starting with a mozzarella slice on the bottom, alternately stack cheese slices and tomato slices, ending up with a tomato slice on the top. Place 3 basil leaves on top of each stack, then put each stack on a chilled plate.

In a large bowl add the vinegar, oil, salt, and pepper, and mix well with a whisk. Pour the dressing over the basil, tomato, and mozzarella stacks and serve.

Good for B and C dieters.

Arugula Salad with Cucumbers, Feta, and Mint

SERVES 2.

4 ounces fresh mint
6 tablespoons macadamia nut oil
2 tablespoons sherry vinegar
Salt
1 medium cucumber
4 radishes, trimmed
5 ounces baby arugula, washed and dried
2 ounces feta cheese, crumbled
Black pepper, freshly ground
12 small black olives (optional)

Coarsely chop the mint leaves and place in a large bowl. Combine them with the oil, vinegar, and salt.

Peel the cucumber and slice lengthwise into very thin slices. Then slice it again into long spaghetti-like strands. Slice the radishes as fine as possible.

In a large bowl add the arugula, cucumber, and radishes. Add the vinegar and oil mixture and toss evenly to coat. Add the feta and black pepper and gently fold them through the salad.

Distribute the salad among the plates, making sure that each plate has some of the ingredients.

Top the salads with olives if desired.

Good for A, B, and C dieters.

Crisp Garden Salad with Herbs, Cherry Tomatoes, and Olives

SERVES 4.

This salad has a Greek feel to it, so if you want to add a little feta cheese, go right ahead. Also, the cherry tomatoes are optional in this salad. This is a perfect summer salad because of all the different ingredients. If some of the ingredients aren't available in your market, however, don't be alarmed. Just buy the freshest ingredients you can.

Juice of 1 lemon
¼ cup macadamia nut oil
Salt
Black pepper, freshly ground
½ cup green cabbage, shredded
1 cup baby arugula, washed and dried
1 cup baby spinach, washed and dried
¼ cup fresh cilantro leaves, washed and dried
¼ cup fresh parsley leaves, washed and dried
5 scallions, white part only, chopped
10 cherry tomatoes (optional)
½ cup green olives, rinsed and drained

Combine the lemon juice, macadamia nut oil, salt, and pepper in a large bowl. Add the rest of the ingredients and toss well. Serve the salad immediately in a large bowl and let your guests fight over it.

Good for A, B, and C dieters.

Warm Frisée Salad with Pine Nuts and Pomegranates

SERVES 4–6.

This salad originated in Granada in southern Spain and is served during the winter months. Granada is the Spanish word for "pomegranate." The thing I like most about this dish is that it can be served as a side vegetable or as a freestanding salad course.

2 large heads frisée, separated, washed, and dried
¼ cup pine nuts
2 small garlic cloves, peeled and crushed
3 tablespoons macadamia nut oil
1 tablespoon aged sherry vinegar
3 teaspoons dry sherry
Salt
White pepper, freshly ground
¾ cup pomegranate seeds

Tear the frisée leaves into 2-inch pieces and place them in a large bowl.

In a medium skillet, lightly toast the pine nuts over medium heat. Remove the pine nuts from the skillet and place them on a warm plate.

Gently warm the garlic in the oil until the garlic is light golden, then discard the garlic, saving the oil. Add the vinegar and dry sherry to the oil and bring just to a boil. Pour this mixture over the greens to warm them. Add the salt, pepper, and pine nuts and toss the salad well. Scatter pomegranate seeds on top and serve at once.

Good for A, B, and C dieters.

Colorful Snow Pea Salad

SERVES 4.

This great recipe was contributed by Gayle Pruitt of Dallas, Texas.

1 red bell pepper
1 orange bell pepper
1 pound snow peas
Lemon and Macadamia Nut Oil Dressing (recipe follows)
½ small red onion, thinly sliced
Grape tomatoes for garnish (optional)
Ripe olives, sliced in half for garnish (optional)
Salt
Black pepper, freshly ground

Slice the red and orange bell peppers into thin julienne slices. Blanch the snow peas in boiling water for 30 seconds, then place in an ice bath. Put the peppers and snow peas in a large bowl and marinate with ½ cup of the dressing for 30 minutes. Arrange the peppers and peas on a platter and scatter the onion slices over the plate. Garnish with tomatoes and olives, if desired. Add salt and pepper to taste. To vary this salad, crumble either 4 ounces of blue cheese or 4 ounces of feta over the salad.

Lemon and Macadamia Nut Oil Dressing
MAKES 1½ CUPS.

There are as many variations on this as your imagination can dream up. One of my favorites is to add garlic and fresh basil, although any fresh herb will do nicely. You might also try a couple of drops of Tabasco sauce to give it more of a Southwestern flair.

1 cup macadamia nut oil
2 tablespoons lemon juice, freshly squeezed
1 teaspoon lemon zest
1 teaspoon salt

Add all the ingredients together in a cruet and let the dressing stand for at least 30 minutes.

You will need only half of the dressing for this particular recipe, and it will keep up to 1 week in the refrigerator, depending on the herbs you choose. If you use dried herbs, the dressing will last longer.

Good for A, B, and C dieters.

Nutty Lemon Vinaigrette

MAKES 1 CUP.

Because you are learning to cook Hamptons style, this is another example of a recipe of which there are an unlimited number of combinations that you can come up with. By using these sauces on a variety of dishes, you can serve different meals all the time, yet hold onto a mere handful of recipes.

Vinaigrettes are sauces as well as dressings. They can be used in a multitude of ways and should not be relegated only to gracing a salad. Think of these as recipes to accompany fish, chicken, meat, and vegetable dishes, as well as salads.

The two key ingredients in vinaigrette are vinegar and oil. Use only the best you can afford of both, and your vinaigrette is guaranteed to be a success.

¼ cup lemon juice, freshly squeezed
¾ cup macadamia nut oil
1 teaspoon kosher salt
1 teaspoon black pepper, freshly ground

In a small bowl, whisk together all the ingredients.

Good for A, B, and C dieters.

Balsamic Vinaigrette

¼ cup aged balsamic vinegar
¾ cup extra-virgin olive oil
½ teaspoon salt
½ teaspoon black pepper, freshly ground
2 tablespoons fresh marjoram, chopped

In a small bowl, whisk together all the ingredients.

Good for A, B, and C dieters.

Cantabrian Vinaigrette

MAKES 1 CUP.

1 small red onion, finely chopped
6 tablespoons red wine vinegar
Pinch salt
Black pepper, freshly ground
1 small clove garlic
4 salt-packed anchovy filets, soaked and squeezed dry
¾ cup macadamia nut oil

Mix the onions with the vinegar in a bowl. Add the salt and dissolve it into the vinegar by stirring with a spoon or whisk. Add the pepper. Separately, pound the garlic and anchovies to a paste in a mortar and add them to the bowl. Whisk in the oil.

Good for A, B, and C dieters.

Cote D'Azur Vinaigrette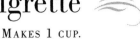

MAKES 1 CUP.

2 large cloves garlic, minced
½ cup red wine vinegar
Pinch salt
Pinch black pepper, freshly ground
1 cup extra-virgin olive oil
¼ cup fresh basil, chopped

Whisk the garlic, vinegar, salt, and pepper together until the salt is well dissolved. Add the oil and basil and whisk until well blended.

Good for A, B, and C dieters.

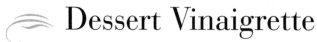

Dessert Vinaigrette

Vinaigrettes are so versatile that they can even be used for dessert dishes. This is great drizzled over a plate of fresh seasonal vegetables, or it can be drizzled over the ice cream or any of the pies in the dessert section of this book for some extra flavor.

¼ cup pomegranate juice
¼ cup teaspoon balsamic vinegar
½ cup estate-bottled extra-virgin olive oil
1 teaspoon walnut oil or macadamia nut oil
Salt
Black pepper, freshly ground

In a small bowl, whisk together all the ingredients.

Good for B and C dieters.

The Miami Beach Vinaigrette

1 tablespoon grapefruit juice
1 tablespoon lime juice
1 tablespoon lemon juice
1 tablespoon orange juice
¼ cup balsamic vinegar
¼ teaspoon kosher salt
½ teaspoon fresh oregano, chopped
¾ cup macadamia nut oil

In a small bowl, using a wire whisk, mix together all the ingredients.

Good for A, B, and C dieters.

Southampton Vinaigrette

MAKES 1 CUP.

2 shallots, finely chopped
Scant ¼ cup sherry vinegar
1 teaspoon dry sherry
1 teaspoon thyme, chopped
Salt
White pepper, freshly ground
¾ cup macadamia nut oil

In a small bowl, whisk together the shallots, vinegar, thyme, a little salt, and pepper and mix well to dissolve the salt. When the salt is dissolved, whisk in the oil.

Good for A, B, and C dieters.

Malaga Vinaigrette

If you have never used champagne vinegar, you are in for a real treat. The flavor is subtle but extravagant and completely delicious.

¾ cup champagne vinegar
¼ cup dry white wine
1 teaspoon Spanish saffron threads
1 small onion, chopped
Salt
Black pepper, freshly ground
1 tablespoon Dijon mustard
1 lemon, zest and juice
1 cup macadamia nut oil

In a small saucepan, combine the vinegar, saffron threads, red onion, salt, and pepper and bring to a boil. Cook over high heat until the liquid is reduced to about one third. Remove from the heat and stir in the mustard, lemon zest, and juice. Place the mixture in a food processor or blender, and, with the motor running, slowly pour the oil in until the mixture is emulsified.

Good for A, B, and C dieters.

Further Lane Vinaigrette

MAKES 1 CUP.

We wanted to add a few recipes to make you gasp. Because of the expense of this dish, you may want to save it for dinner guests whom you really want to impress. If you have never been lucky enough to eat truffles, their flavor is very earthy and sublime—you don't need a lot of them to make a big taste splash.

3 tablespoons black truffles, fresh or canned, thinly sliced
Salt
Black pepper, freshly ground
¼ cup aged sherry vinegar
¾ cup macadamia nut oil

Place the black truffles, salt, pepper, and vinegar in a large bowl and whisk together. After they're combined, slowly whisk in the oil.

Good for A, B, and C dieters.

Madras Vinaigrette

¼ cup champagne vinegar
2 tablespoons coriander seeds
Salt
Black pepper, freshly ground
2 tablespoons lemon juice
2 tablespoons lemon zest
¾ cup macadamia nut oil

Whisk together the first six ingredients in a large bowl. Then slowly add the oil and whisk together well.

Good for A, B, and C dieters.

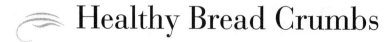

Healthy Bread Crumbs

1 loaf healthy whole-grain bread

To make whole wheat bread crumbs, spelt breadcrumbs, or even sprouted bread crumbs, simply allow the bread to get stale or, better yet, place the slices in a 250°F oven for 15 minutes on a flat cookie sheet, checking and turning them over every few minutes to make sure they don't burn.

If you need only a small amount of bread crumbs, you can toast the bread in a toaster for the same effect. When the slices are fully dried or toasted, remove them from the oven and allow them to cool. Break them up, put them in a food processor, and pulse until you have the bread crumb consistency that you desire. At this point, you can divide the crumbs, season them in different ways, and save them for when you need them. I am always a big fan of making a lot and saving the extra for another day. These will store for months in the freezer. You can make them with Italian seasonings, Indian style, or in any way you desire. They will easily spice up your meals without becoming boring or redundant.

Good for A, B, and C dieters.

Couscous Stuffing

This can be used as a stuffing for turkey or as a side dish any time of the year. Besides, who doesn't admit that the stuffing is his or her favorite part of Thanksgiving?

1 box 5-minute whole-grain couscous
16 ounces organic chicken broth
3 tablespoons macadamia nut oil
1 small onion, finely chopped
½ cup celery, finely chopped
¼ teaspoon poultry seasoning
Dash sage
Salt
Black pepper, freshly ground

Follow the directions on the box of couscous, using the chicken broth instead of water and using 1 tablespoon of macadamia nut oil instead of butter. In a separate skillet, sauté the onions and celery with 2 tablespoons of the oil for 3 to 5 minutes—don't let them brown. Add the onions and celery to the cooked couscous and mix through. Add the poultry seasoning and sage. Fluff the couscous with a fork. Add salt and pepper to taste. With this recipe, you can add almost any herb your family likes. Even mushrooms can be thrown in; they should be sautéed with the onions and the celery.

Good for B and C dieters.

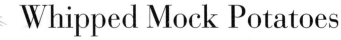

Whipped Mock Potatoes

SERVES 4–6.

This is one of my favorite recipes. It is a great way to get kids to eat vegetables without their realizing it. I've used this same recipe for broccoli, and it also tastes great. I've used a similar recipe for many years, but I must admit that my friend the great chef Tom Valenti helped me hone this one for a truly special treat.

1 head cauliflower
¼ cup butter, softened
2 tablespoons macadamia nut oil
8 ounces sour cream
2 ounces Parmesan cheese, grated
Salt
Black pepper, freshly ground

Preheat the oven to 400°F.

Steam the cauliflower until it's very tender. Drain and then spread the florets on a baking sheet. Bake for 10 to 12 minutes. Remove the cookie sheet from the oven and, using a potato masher, mash the cauliflower well. Return it to the oven for 10 more minutes. The more you dry out the cauliflower, the more like potatoes it will be. Remove the cauliflower from the oven and put it into a blender or food processor. Add the butter, oil, and sour cream to the processor and blend until it reaches the desired consistency. Add the Parmesan cheese and salt and pepper to taste.

Good for A, B, and C dieters.

Pan-Roasted Cauliflower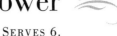

SERVES 6.

Roasting is Jeff's favorite way of preparing vegetables. Roasting vegetables allows the sugars to caramelize, creating a sweetness and an earthiness that are difficult to obtain with other cooking methods.

1 head cauliflower
2 tablespoons macadamia nut oil
Kosher salt
White pepper, freshly ground
1 tablespoon fresh thyme
1 tablespoon unsalted butter
Pinch nutmeg, freshly ground

Trim the cauliflower into 1-inch florets. Place a large skillet over medium-high heat and add the oil. When the oil is hot but not smoking, add the florets, salt, pepper, and thyme. Cook the cauliflower until the florets begin to color, about 7 minutes, tossing them frequently. Add the butter and continue cooking until the cauliflower is tender and light brown, about 5 minutes. Grate some nutmeg over the cauliflower. Drain the cauliflower on paper towels and serve.

Good for A, B, and C dieters.

Cheddar Cauliflower

SERVES 6.

This recipe was sent to me by Jennifer T. Her kids hated vegetables until I recommended that she smother them with cheese. My mother tried this trick with me, and it has worked ever since. This recipe can also be used with broccoli. I would also offer this to husbands who won't eat their vegetables.

1 head cauliflower, cut into florets
3 tablespoons macadamia nut oil
1½ cups heavy cream
⅔ cup cheddar cheese, shredded
1 teaspoon salt
½ teaspoon black pepper, freshly ground
6 strips bacon, cooked and crumbled

Preheat the oven to 350°F.

Steam the cauliflower for about 10 minutes or until crisp-tender. Place it on a greased baking sheet. In a heavy saucepan, heat the oil and gradually add the cream over medium heat, whisking continuously until it's bubbly. Add the cheese and seasonings until the mixture starts to thicken or you can use one of the vegetable or guar gums as a thickening agent. Because there is no flour in this recipe, you may have to cook off a lot of the cream until you get the desired thickness. Pour this mixture over the cauliflower and bake for 25 minutes. Top with crumbled bacon and serve.

Good for A, B, and C dieters.

Oven-Roasted Beets

SERVES 6–8.

20 medium beets
¼ cup macadamia nut oil
Kosher salt
Black pepper, freshly ground
¼ cup extra-virgin olive oil

Preheat the oven to 350°F. Wash the beets under cold running water. Trim the greens and bottoms from the beets.

Combine the beets and macadamia nut oil in a large bowl. Season with salt and pepper and toss to coat. Transfer the beets to a large roasting pan and cover with aluminum foil. Roast until the beets can be easily pierced with a knife, about 40 minutes. Let the beets cool for about 5 minutes, then peel them gently, using a clean dish towel. Cut the beets into quarters. Toss them with the olive oil and add salt and pepper if needed.

Serve immediately.

Good for A, B, and C dieters.

Pan-Roasted Carrots

SERVES 6–8.

25–30 baby carrots or 3 large carrots cut into 3- to 4-inch-long strips
2 tablespoons macadamia nut oil
Kosher salt
Black pepper, freshly ground
1 tablespoon unsalted butter
1 sprig fresh thyme

Peel the carrots, then trim them, leaving on an inch or so of the green tops. Heat a large skillet over medium heat. Add the oil and when it's hot, add the carrots. Season with salt and pepper. Sauté the carrots so they turn golden brown on all sides, about 5 minutes. Add the butter and thyme and continue cooking for about 5 minutes or until tender. Drain the carrots on paper towels before serving.

Good for A, B, and C dieters.

Confetti Coleslaw

I love a great warm coleslaw, and this is it. This is another basic recipe that may be used with various vegetables, according to the season, to make many different dishes. It was sent by a colleague from Dallas, whom I will name later on in the book. This dish is excellent with grilled dishes and even delicious in the winter when cabbage is in season.

2–3 pounds fresh cabbage, red or green or in combination
1 large green bell pepper
1 large red bell pepper
1 large orange or yellow bell pepper
1 red onion
½ cup macadamia nut oil
1 cup cider vinegar
1 teaspoon salt
1 teaspoon mustard powder
1 teaspoon celery seed

Trim and wash the cabbage, bell peppers, and onion. Cut them into chunks and add to a food processor in batches, pulsing until the vegetables are the size of large pieces of confetti. If you don't have a food processor, finely chop the vegetables with a knife.

Transfer the vegetables to a large, heatproof glass bowl. Put the remaining ingredients in a medium saucepan over medium-high heat. Bring to a boil, then pour the hot liquid over the vegetables. Place the bowl in a preheated 375°F oven for 20 minutes or until the vegetables are fully wilted. If you prefer a cold slaw, instead of cooking this, place the bowl in the refrigerator and serve the cole slaw chilled.

Good for B and C dieters.

Fall Vegetable Medley

SERVES 6–8.

Menestras de verduras, or vegetable stews, are made throughout Spain in conjunction with the seasons. The dish changes depending on the time of the year. Jeff has given us two versions of this dish, so that you can see what it's like to simply change the ingredients without changing the steps for cooking the dish. Use the freshest vegetables available, and make sure they are in season. Seasonality is key. Following is a list of fall vegetables that Jeff likes to use, but you can omit some or add others as you wish, depending on the vegetables your family likes to eat. Jeff prefers to blanch the vegetables, but you can steam them if you want.

½ pound broccoli florets
½ pound cauliflower florets
½ pound brussels sprouts
1 red onion, peeled and quartered
2 medium carrots, peeled and quartered
½ acorn squash, seeded and diced
2 garlic cloves, minced
¼ cup macadamia nut oil
Coarse sea salt

Bring 5 quarts of salted water to a rapid boil. Cook each vegetable individually for 1 minute. Then rinse them under cold water for about 1 minute to stop the cooking process.

In a large skillet heat 2 tablespoons of oil over medium heat. Add the garlic and sauté for 1 minute until lightly golden. Add the vegetables and cook for about 5 minutes until heated through, stirring occasionally. Place them on a warm serving platter and pour the remaining 2 tablespoons of oil over them. Season with coarse sea salt.

Good for A, B, and C dieters.

Summer Vegetable Medley

This recipe follows the same steps as in the previous recipe but uses different seasonal vegetables.

½ pound green beans
½ pound yellow beans
½ pound asparagus, bottom quarter trimmed
½ pound snow peas
½ pound spring onions, quartered
½ pound fennel, quartered
2 garlic cloves, minced
¼ cup macadamia nut oil
Coarse sea salt

Follow the directions as for the Fall Vegetable Medley recipe.

Good for A, B, and C dieters.

Green Beans with Shallots

SERVES 8.

Jenna D. sent me this recipe from Chicago. She likes to serve this dish at Thanksgiving instead of the more traditional recipe that uses canned soup and other unhealthy ingredients. She was nervous about serving it the first year, but now her guests ask for this recipe more than any other.

2 pounds fresh green beans, trimmed
2 medium shallots, diced
1 tablespoon macadamia nut oil
1 teaspoon fresh thyme
1 teaspoon fresh rosemary
1 teaspoon fines herbes
Black pepper, freshly ground

Cook the green beans in a large pot of boiling salted water for about 8 minutes. Drain the beans and put them in an ice bath to stop the cooking process. Remove from the ice bath and drain. In a medium frying pan over medium-high heat, sauté the shallots in the oil for about 3 minutes or until lightly browned. Add the green beans and herbs, season with pepper to taste, and serve.

Good for A, B, and C dieters.

Vegetable Cheese Medley

You are probably noticing a theme running through the recipes that my patients or I contribute. Jeff is much more adventurous with vegetables, but for most of us, a good bit of cheese can make almost any vegetable edible. Here is a recipe sent to us from one of my favorite patients, who has lost 84 pounds as of this writing.

½ cup macadamia nut oil
2 cups baby carrots
2 cups broccoli florets
2 cups cauliflower florets
2 garlic cloves, minced
1 medium onion, chopped
1 cup mozzarella cheese, shredded
½ cup Parmesan cheese, shredded
¾ teaspoon black pepper, freshly ground

Preheat the oven to 350°F.

Heat the oil in a large skillet over medium-high heat until it's just below its smoke point. Add all the vegetables except the onions and sauté for about 10 minutes. Add the garlic and onion and sauté for an additional 5 minutes.

In a 2-quart greased baking dish, spread out the vegetable mixture evenly. Mix the cheeses together in a separate bowl, then sprinkle them over the vegetables, and season with pepper. Bake for 25 minutes. For a crispier crust, about 5 minutes before the vegetables are fully cooked, add an additional layer of Parmesan cheese and place the dish under the broiler for 4 minutes.

Good for A, B, and C dieters.

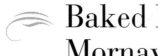

Baked Broccoli with Mornay Sauce

SERVES 8.

Mornay Sauce is really easy to make and can help disguise the taste of vegetables. Vegetables, especially cruciferous ones like broccoli and cauliflower, produce a chemical that is extremely cancer-protective, so I try to find ways to encourage you and your family to eat them. This recipe can also be made with cauliflower.

Salt
1 pound broccoli
Mornay Sauce (see recipe, page 61)
Parmesan cheese to taste

Preheat the oven to 350°F.

Bring 2 quarts of salted water to a boil over high heat. Place the broccoli florets in the water and cook for 5 minutes. Strain them, put them in a baking dish, and cover with Mornay Sauce.

Cook for 30 minutes until the sauce is bubbly and the broccoli is very soft. Remove from the heat, turn the oven to broil, and sprinkle the dish with Parmesan cheese. Place the dish under the broiler for an additional 5 minutes to create a crispy top that the entire family will fight over.

Good for A, B, and C dieters.

Oven-Fried Broccoli

SERVES 8.

This recipe was sent by another harried mom who couldn't get vegetables into her child's diet. She discovered this trick, and now the child wants to eat it every night. Carla has done this with cauliflower, asparagus, and even eggplant.

1 cup maconnaise (see recipe, page 73)
1 head broccoli, broken into florets
1 cup pork rinds, crushed

Preheat the oven to 350°F.

In a large bowl, add the maconnaise and broccoli and stir to coat well. Or, put these ingredients in a ziplock bag and shake it to get the same effect. Spread out the broccoli on a greased cookie sheet, and then pour the pork rinds onto the broccoli. Toss until the broccoli is covered on both sides. Bake for 1 hour. Depending on the vegetable you use, the cooking time will vary.

Good for A, B, and C dieters.

Swiss Chard Rounds

SERVES 8.

This recipe was sent to me by the chef of a very famous motion picture director. While I was writing this book, I sent an e-mail out to all of my patients, asking them to contribute recipes. Not only did that make it easier for Jeff and me to write this book, but, more important, it allows you to see that anyone can cook and the recipes don't have to be fancy to be included in a cookbook. This chef lost 34 pounds eating delicious recipes like this one.

1½ pounds Swiss chard, cleaned and well drained
Macadamia nut oil spray
6 strips bacon, diced
1 cup leeks, finely diced
5 cloves garlic, peeled and minced
Salt
Black pepper, freshly ground
½ cup cashew butter
4 eggs, separated
⅛ teaspoon nutmeg
2 ounces Parmesan cheese, grated

Preheat the oven to 375°F.

Separate the stems from leaves of the Swiss chard and chop each separately. Spray six 6-ounce muffin tins with the macadamia nut oil.

Put the bacon in a heavy skillet over low heat. When the bacon turns golden, add the chard stems, leeks, and garlic. Season with salt and pepper and cook over low heat until the vegetables are tender but not brown. Transfer to a bowl.

Add the chopped chard leaves to the skillet, increase the heat to medium high, and cook until the chard leaves are wilted. Add the leaves to the bowl and mix in the cashew butter and egg yolks. In a separate bowl, beat the egg whites with an electric mixer until they hold a peak but are still somewhat creamy. Fold them into the other mixture, reseason with salt and pepper, and add the nutmeg.

Pour the mixture in the prepared muffin tins and bake for 15 minutes. Then sprinkle Parmesan cheese on top and put the muffin tins back in the oven for 5 more minutes. Remove the tins from the oven, unmold the rounds, and serve hot.

Good for A, B, and C dieters.

Spaghetti Squash

SERVES 4.

This recipe was sent to me by a patient who said that he could almost imagine it was just like Sunday afternoons, sitting down in front of the television set and watching football with a bowl of "spaghetti." James Z. lost 75 pounds following the Hamptons Diet regimen.

1 large spaghetti squash
¼ cup macadamia nut oil
¼ cup organic butter
¼ cup grated Parmesan cheese
Salt
Black pepper, freshly ground

Place the spaghetti squash on a baking sheet in a preheated 400°F oven. Bake for 45 minutes or until the squash is soft to the touch with an oven mitt. Remove the squash from the oven and let it sit for 10 to 15 minutes. Split the squash in half and remove the seeds. Put on an oven mitt and hold the squash over a mixing bowl. Using a fork, shred both halves of the squash out of its skin into the bowl. You'll see why it's called spaghetti squash. As it shreds, you'll notice the long spaghettilike strands. Add the macadamia nut oil and mix the butter through the squash as it melts. Add the Parmesan cheese and give the squash a quick mix. Add salt and pepper to taste.

Good for A, B, and C dieters.

Whipped Sweet Potatoes Southern Style

This recipe was sent to us by Martie Whittekin from Dallas.

3 large sweet potatoes, cooked
2 ounces Southern Comfort
8-ounce package mascarpone, softened (Italian cream cheese)
½ cup whipping cream
2 or 3 small packets stevia (available in most health and
    natural food stores)

Using a hand mixer or potato masher, whip the sweet potatoes with the Southern Comfort and softened mascarpone cheese until the mixture is smooth. In a separate cold stainless steel bowl, beat the whipping cream, with a hand mixer, until it's stiff. Add the stevia when the whipping cream is almost ready. Add a little of the whipping cream to the sweet potato mixture and beat it. Then fold the remaining whipping cream into the sweet potato mixture, which should now be light and fluffy.

Good for B and C dieters.

Roasted Zucchini with Feta and Mint

SERVES 4.

Ella T. sent me this recipe from New Orleans. I have not heard from her since the Hurricane Katrina disaster, but I certainly hope she is well. I wanted to honor her by including this recipe in the book. The last time we spoke, she had lost 32 pounds.

2 yellow zucchini, cut into 1-inch cubes
2 green zucchini, cut into 1-inch cubes
3 tablespoons macadamia nut oil
Salt
Black pepper, freshly ground
¼ cup feta cheese, crumbled
2 tablespoons fresh mint, chopped (from the garden, if possible)
Lemon wedges for garnish (optional)

Preheat the oven to 450°F.

Spread out the zucchini on a baking sheet and drizzle with the macadamia nut oil; add a pinch of salt and the black pepper. Bake for about 40 minutes or until the zucchini is a light brown. Stir it once or twice and be sure not to overcook. Toss the zucchini with the feta, mint, and more salt and pepper. Put it on a serving plate and garnish with the lemon wedges, if desired, for a more colorful presentation. This dish can be served hot or warm.

Good for A, B, and C dieters.

Fennel and Pear with Parmigiano Reggiano and Balsamic Glaze

Serves 2.

This dish is an old family favorite that I learned from grandmother DiCapprio. It is truly a wonderful appetizer full of bright flavors.

½ cup balsamic vinegar
½ pound Parmigiano Reggiano cheese, shaved into long strips
½ cup of fennel bulbs, shaved into thin strips
1 organic Bosc pear, sliced
Black pepper, freshly ground

In a saucepan, reduce the balsamic vinegar by half, until it is almost thick in consistency. Divide the cheese and fennel strips between two plates, placing them in a pile in the center of each plate. Arrange half of the pear around each cheese and fennel pile. Drizzle a small amount of the reduced balsamic vinegar over the cheese, fennel, and pear on each plate. Top each dish with black pepper.

Good for A, B, and C dieters.

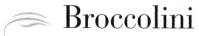

Broccolini

SERVES 2.

This is a wonderful side dish. Broccolini resembles broccoli rabe, but is not bit-
ter and has an almost sweet buttery flavor.

Macadamia nut oil
2 cloves garlic, thinly sliced
1 pound broccolini
¼ cup slivered almonds, toasted
Salt
Black pepper, freshly ground
½ cup organic chicken broth

Pour enough macadamia nut oil into a cast-iron skillet to cover the bottom.
Add the garlic and lightly sauté just until it starts to turn golden. Add the
broccolini to the skillet and continue to sauté. Pour the chicken broth into the
skillet and cook, covered, for about 10 minutes. Remove the cover and sauté
until the broth has cooked off. Add the toasted almonds. Salt and pepper to
taste and serve.

Good for A, B, and C dieters.

7

Entertaining the Hamptons Diet Way

To most of us who go to the Hamptons, entertaining at home is one of life's biggest pleasures. Keep in mind that most New Yorkers have small apartments and tiny kitchens back in the city, where we spend most of our time, so to actually have the space to host guests is exhilarating. Therefore, we take full advantage of the opportunity to entertain. The Hamptons are filled with fresh food and produce—farms, farm stands, the freshest fish—why go out to dinner? Leave the restaurant scene to the glitterati. True Hamptonites stay home, cook, and entertain.

These next few recipes may not seem like elegant entertaining ideas, but, let me tell you, the best entertaining ideas are always the simplest. Most adults would rather act like children when it comes to food, but we're too sophisticated to admit this to anyone other than the people we love the most. Even then, we are sometimes closet eaters.

I learned how to entertain from one of the grandes dames of the New York social circuit, who recently passed away, and the most important thing she ever taught me was to always keep the guests a little off guard. Give them a little of what they expect and a lot of what they don't. It's worked for me over the years, and it will soon have you being the hostess or host with je ne sais quoi. Make it fun for yourself, and it will be fun for your guests, too.

Besides, I've found that it's customary now to bring children to many events, whereas a few years ago this was unheard of. Having families dine together requires a good host or hostess to compose the menu a little differently, but you don't have to turn your home into a diner, offering multiple choices to everyone. I think the recipes in this section will provide you with everything you need for the perfect dinner party or reception. Everything but the guests, and when the word gets out about your culinary creations, they will be lining up to get invited to your parties.

These recipes can each be made far ahead of time and served cool or reheated, and they are portable, too. This is a great way of always having snacks on hand for your kids or any unexpected guests.

Chicken Fingers avec Fresh Herbs

These are nothing more than flavorful chicken fingers without the breading, with adult tastes and textures that make them fun for an afternoon party after the beach or with drinks before dinner.

¼ cup lemon juice, freshly squeezed
2 tablespoons macadamia nut oil
1 tablespoon fresh thyme, chopped
1 tablespoon fresh rosemary, chopped
1 tablespoon fresh parsley, chopped
1 clove garlic, minced
Salt
Black pepper, freshly ground
1 pound chicken breasts, skinless, boneless,
    cut into finger-size pieces
1 cup macadamia nut oil

Mix all the ingredients except for the cup of macadamia nut oil in a large ziplock bag, and let marinate for several hours or overnight in the refrigerator. Heat the cup of oil in a medium-size skillet until it's very hot. Remove the chicken fingers from the marinade and sauté over medium heat until lightly browned. Remove them from the heat and place on a dish covered in paper towels to drain. They're best served at room temperature with one of the many tasty dips that follow.

Good for A, B, and C dieters.

Breaded Chicken Fingers

SERVES 8.

This recipe does call for bread crumbs, so please refer to page 174 to learn how to make healthy crumbs. Never use store-bought crumbs unless you can be certain they are made with whole-grain flour.

2 tablespoons lemon juice, freshly squeezed

2 teaspoons Worcestershire sauce

1 teaspoon paprika

1 teaspoon salt

1 teaspoon black pepper, freshly ground

½ teaspoon garlic powder

1 pound chicken breasts, skinless, boneless, cut into finger-size pieces

1 tablespoon macadamia nut oil

½ pound dried whole-grain bread crumbs, finely pulverized in
   food processor

In a large bowl, mix all the ingredients except the breadcrumbs well. Transfer to a large ziplock bag and let marinate for several hours or overnight in the refrigerator.

Preheat the oven to 350°F.

Drain the chicken fingers and roll them in the bread crumbs. Discard any juices that may be in the bag, as they are contaminated by the uncooked chicken. Grease a baking sheet with additional macadamia nut oil. Place the chicken fingers on the baking sheet and bake for about 20 to 25 minutes or until lightly browned and cooked through. These are best served at room temperature with a dipping sauce.

Good for A, B, and C dieters.

Asian Chicken Tenders

This is another variation on the same theme, to keep it always interesting and never boring. That is my least-favorite thing to hear, as a physician who specializes in nutrition. How can nutrition be boring when there are so many foods and spices to choose from? Get creative, folks!

1 pound chicken breasts, skinless, boneless, cut into
    finger-size pieces
1 cup heavy cream
1 tablespoon sesame seed oil
2 tablespoons lemon juice, freshly squeezed
1 clove garlic, minced
1 teaspoon Worcestershire sauce
2 tablespoons soy sauce
1 teaspoon paprika
½ teaspoon cayenne pepper
1 teaspoon salt
1 teaspoon black pepper, freshly ground
4 cups soft whole-grain bread crumbs (see recipe, page 174)
¾ cup sesame seeds
¼ cup macadamia nut oil

Combine the chicken with the next ten ingredients in a large ziplock bag and let marinate for several hours or overnight in the refrigerator.

When you're ready to prepare the chicken, preheat the oven to 350°F.

Drain the chicken and discard the juices. Combine the bread crumbs and sesame seeds in a large bowl or high-sided dish. Add the chicken and toss to coat. Place it on a lightly greased cookie sheet sprayed with macadamia nut oil and brush with the macadamia nut oil. Bake for about 30 minutes. These chicken tenders can be served warm or at room temperature.

Good for A, B, and C dieters.

Chicken-Fried Steak Fingers

SERVES 8.

I was really excited when I saw this recipe. I thought I'd never be able to eat chicken-fried steak again. For those of us who grew up in the North, this is a rare and very indulgent treat. I lived in Dallas for five years, and people didn't think twice about eating this food. There never seemed to be any guilt about it. Perhaps it's because those of us in the Northeast are more neurotic; I don't know. All I do know is that I asked Jeff to try to turn this into a healthy dish. First he laughed at me. Then I was surprised when I found this recipe sitting in my e-mail inbox!

1 egg
1 cup heavy cream
1 pound top round steak, cut into ½-inch strips
1 cup soy flour*
½ cup macadamia nut oil
Salt
Black pepper, freshly ground

Beat the egg and cream together in a small bowl. Coat the strips of steak with flour, dip in the egg mixture, then recoat with flour. Pour the oil into a skillet and heat it over medium heat until just below its smoke point. Place the steak in the skillet and fry until the coating is brown and crispy. Remove the steak to paper towels and add salt and pepper to taste immediately. These steak fingers are best served hot.

Good for A, B, and C dieters.

*Jeff made this recipe with soy flour, but the dish can also be made with any whole-grain flour, including brown rice, buckwheat, spelt, amaranth, and so on. The trick is to know that the oil must be extra hot, or the coating will come off in the skillet.

Sauces and Dips

Dips and sauces can be used for a variety of dishes. They can be poured on all of the previous chicken finger recipes or they can marinate ribs for grilling. They can be used to dip vegetables into, or they can be basted on chicken parts and baked in the oven. Dips and sauces can turn a boring meal into an adventure.

I didn't really learn about sauces and that there was such a thing as a sauce chef until I worked with Alison Becker Hurt, my friend who owns the restaurant where Jeff is the chef. She taught me many things about the fine art of dining. When visiting the Hamptons, be sure to eat at the restaurant Alison in Bridgehampton, New York. Call ahead first, though; it is always booked.

The thing that separates chefs from cooks is the sauce. Never get too heavy-handed because that can destroy a great meal, but don't be afraid of spices. Allow your family and guests to try different flavor combinations. These sauces and dips can really entice your kids to eat healthy. Put the sauces on everything you can think of but especially on vegetables to tempt children's still-developing palates. Have fun with these!

Plum Sauce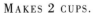

MAKES 2 CUPS.

1½ cups red plum jam, sugar-free and all-fruit only
1½ teaspoons mustard
1 teaspoon horseradish
1½ teaspoons lemon juice, freshly squeezed

Mix all the ingredients in a small saucepan and bring to a boil over medium heat. Remove the sauce from the heat and pour it into a bowl. Let chill in the refrigerator for at least 1 hour before using it.

Good for A, B, and C dieters, depending on the portion size.

Spicy Plum Island Sauce

MAKES 2 CUPS.

1½ cups plum jam, sugar-free and all-fruit only
2 tablespoons white wine vinegar
1 tablespoon Splenda or lo-han
1 tablespoon onion, dried, minced
1 teaspoon red pepper flakes, crushed
1 clove garlic, minced
½ teaspoon ground ginger

In a saucepan over medium heat, combine all the ingredients and bring to a boil, stirring constantly. Remove the sauce from the heat and set it aside. This sauce may be served warm or cold.

Depending on the portion size, this sauce can be good for A, B, and C dieters.

Peacock Sauce Southern Style

1 cup chicken broth
¼ cup peanuts, shelled, skinned, fresh roasted
1 tablespoon lemon juice, freshly squeezed
1 tablespoon fresh ginger, minced
¼ teaspoon cayenne pepper
1 garlic clove, minced
Salt

Mix the first six ingredients in a blender or food processor until smooth, about 1 minute. Transfer the mixture to a saucepan. Over medium-low heat, simmer, stirring constantly, until it's thick enough to coat a spoon, about 10 minutes. Season with salt to taste. This sauce may be served hot or cold.

Good for A, B, and C dieters.

Balinese Peanut Sauce

MAKES 2 CUPS.

This is a variation on the previous sauce—it tastes wildly different, though. Another variation would be to change the nut that you use, in case you have any guests or people in your household who are allergic to peanuts. I'm sure this recipe would work just as well with cashews, macadamia nuts, almonds, or even walnuts. If you're having a dinner party, make these sauces a few different ways, and watch your guests go wild.

Same ingredients as the previous recipe, plus:

4 teaspoons lo-han or 4 packets stevia
2 tablespoons soy sauce
1 tablespoon fresh cilantro, chopped

Mix all the ingredients except the sweetener, soy sauce, and cilantro in a food processor or blender until smooth, about 1 minute. Transfer the mixture to a saucepan. Before heating it, add the sweetener and soy sauce. Over medium-low heat, simmer until you have achieved the desired consistency, then add the cilantro and remove the sauce from the heat. Let this sauce cool slightly before serving it.

Good for A, B, and C dieters.

Springs Picante Dip

MAKES 2 CUPS.

As many of my patients and readers know, I like things hot and spicy. I asked Jeff to provide a few recipes that could really turn up the heat in the kitchen. Spicy foods are great antiviral and antibacterial agents, so I tend to like these dishes most in the winter.

1 package cream cheese or queso blanco, softened
¼ cup sour cream
1 cup hot or mild Mexican salsa

In a medium-sized bowl, mix the softened cheese and sour cream together with a hand mixer until fully combined. Add the salsa and mix it through the cheeses. Let the dip refrigerate for at least 1 hour before using it to allow for the spiciness to take hold.

Good for A, B, and C dieters.

Indonesian Dipping Sauce

MAKES 2 CUPS.

Indonesia used to be one of my favorite haunts. I have chosen not to travel there because of my political views, but I clearly remember the freshness of the food, especially the fruit that was served on the beaches by wonderful women who used to carry the fruit on their heads. They had just picked the fruit, and they would sit down with you, cut it up, and share it with you. It was a magnificent time in my life, and this recipe is inspired by that era.

5 apricot halves
2 peach halves, canned in their own juice
3 tablespoons Asian plum sauce, or plum fruit-only jam
   (available in any Asian market)
½ red onion, chopped
1 teaspoon mustard powder
¼ cup fresh ginger, minced
Juice of 1 lime, freshly squeezed
1 tablespoon red pepper flakes, crushed
1 garlic clove, minced
3 tablespoons fresh cilantro, minced

Puree all the ingredients except one apricot half and the cilantro in a blender or food processor. Put the dip in a sauce dish and garnish with the cilantro and remaining apricot. If used as a dipping sauce, this is best served cold. The sauce can be used for a barbecue or for roasted chicken, too. I also like it on fresh pork roast. Because it's so versatile, though, you can use this sauce on anything you wish. It would be great on a meaty fish, like brook trout or mackerel, too.

Good for C dieters.

Mount Fuji Dipping Sauce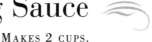

This can be not only a dipping sauce but a great marinade for a pork loin as well.

1½ cups Fuji apples
3 tablespoons soy sauce
¾ cup daikon (Asian white radish), grated
½ teaspoon ground ginger
2 tablespoons mustard powder

Mix all the ingredients in a food processor or blender until the apples are soft but not thoroughly pureed into applesauce. Transfer the ingredients to a saucepan and, over low heat, heat them through. This sauce is best served warm.

Good for A, B, and C dieters.

Wasabi Spiced Dipping Sauce

MAKES 2 CUPS.

I am a frequent visitor to Japan, where I consult with many health companies. On one of my trips there, I mentioned that I really liked wasabi with my sashimi. They asked whether I had ever had true wasabi. I said that I live in New York, where they have the best of everything. So, a few days later, when I was leaving the country, I was presented with a true wasabi root, which looks like a rather ugly ginger root, and a bamboo tool with sharkskin on one side, which is how the Japanese chef grates the wasabi into dishes. Now I can't cook without fresh wasabi. I caution that wasabi root is extremely expensive, however, so for this recipe, the green powder that we're all familiar with will do just fine.

1 cup soy sauce
1 cup rice vinegar
¼ cup wasabi powder
1 teaspoon fresh chives, chopped

In a small bowl, using a whisk, mix all the ingredients. Allow at least a half hour for the wasabi's heat to reach its maximal effect before you serve the sauce.

Good for A, B, and C dieters.

Italian "Gravy" Dipping Sauce

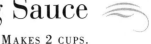

MAKES 2 CUPS.

As a boy, I always called marinara sauce gravy. I think it's something every Italian American experiences, at least in the Northeast. I don't think I learned it wasn't gravy until I was a teenager when I visited a friend's house for dinner.

For me, this sauce can be used for just about anything: calamari, mozzarella cheese, chicken, and so on. There is nothing a good red sauce doesn't complement.

1 tablespoon macadamia nut oil
2 cloves garlic, chopped
5 tomatoes, peeled and finely chopped
1 packet stevia
¼ cup water
2 teaspoons fresh basil, chopped
Salt
Black pepper, freshly ground

In a large skillet, heat the oil. Add the garlic and sauté until light brown and softened, about 8 minutes. Stir in the tomatoes, stevia, water, basil, salt, and pepper. Bring the contents to a boil and cover the skillet. Simmer the sauce over low heat for approximately 45 minutes, stirring occasionally. With this recipe, you are reducing the water, including the water that is naturally found in the tomatoes, so cook it until it reaches the desired consistency. This sauce is best served warm.

Good for B and C dieters.

Blue Cheese Dipping Sauce

MAKES 2 CUPS.

Of course, you can use regular store-bought mayonnaise in this or in any recipe that calls for maconnaise. I just like to make my dishes as healthy as they can be.

¼ pound blue cheese, such as Roquefort or Gorgonzola
½ cup maconnaise (see recipe, page 73)
½ cup sour cream
1 tablespoon lemon juice, freshly squeezed
1 tablespoon wine vinegar
Hot pepper sauce, several dashes to taste

In a small bowl, mash the blue cheese, leaving some small lumps. Whisk in the maconnaise until blended. Add the remaining ingredients and whisk them to blend well. Cover the bowl and refrigerate until serving time.

Good for A, B, and C dieters.

Holiday Latkes

These are so good and, by my standards, better than the original potato latkes. This recipe was given to me by my Hamptons friend and mentor Fran Gare.

4 cups celery root, peeled and grated
2 eggs, lightly beaten
1 medium onion, sliced thin
1 heaping teaspoon sea salt
½ teaspoon white pepper
¼ cup macadamia nut oil
Sour cream, to serve

Mix the celery root, eggs, onion, salt, and pepper together in a medium-sized bowl.

Pour the macadamia nut oil into a skillet and tilt the skillet until the oil coats the bottom. Heat on high until very hot. Carefully drop the celery root mixture by tablespoonfuls into the hot oil. Allow each latke to brown on one side, turn with a slotted spatula, and brown on the other side. Remove to a brown paper bag or paper towels to drain. Serve the latkes with sour cream.

Good for A, B, and C dieters.

Roasted Red Peppers with Anchovies

SERVES 6–8.

Sixty percent of the world's anchovies are caught off the northern coast of Spain. Jeff lived in this region of Spain for about four years and learned how to prepare anchovies in a thousand different ways. This is one of his favorites and is also one of the easiest. As is often the case when cooking, the trick is to use the best-quality anchovies you can find and the heaviest red peppers available.

4 large red bell peppers
¼ cup macadamia nut oil
Salt
4 whole anchovies, salt-packed
10 fresh basil leaves
Black pepper, freshly ground

Preheat the oven to 450°F.

Toss the bell peppers with half the macadamia nut oil and a pinch of salt. Place the peppers on a baking sheet and put them in the oven for about 10 to 15 minutes, turning them over once. The peppers are done when they're slightly charred. Remove from the oven and place in a large bowl. Cover the bowl with plastic wrap and let it sit for about 10 minutes.

Remove the peppers from the bowl, cut them in half lengthwise, and remove the seeds, fibers, and stems. Scrape the charred skin from the peppers with a blunt knife, a paper towel, or your fingers. Put the peppers in a dish and cover with the remaining macadamia nut oil.

Fillet the anchovies and rinse them thoroughly in cold water. Add the anchovy fillets and the basil leaves to the peppers. Season lightly with freshly ground black pepper and gently toss the ingredients, making sure everything is well coated with the oil. Arrange the dish and let marinate in the fridge for about 1 hour before serving.

Good for A, B, and C dieters.

Hard-Boiled Quail Eggs
with Cumin

SERVES 12.

Quail eggs are eaten quite frequently throughout Spain. Traditionally, they are eaten fried and sprinkled with cumin, but for entertaining purposes, Jeff thought that quail eggs hard-boiled and tossed in cumin would be fun and different.

2 dozen quail eggs
2 tablespoons white wine vinegar
2 teaspoons sea salt
2 teaspoons cumin seeds, toasted

In a large stockpot, bring 8 quarts of salted water to a brisk boil. Pour in the vinegar. Gently drop in the quail eggs and boil for 4 minutes. Remove from the pot and let cool.

Toast the cumin seeds in a dry sauté pan for about 2 minutes over medium heat until they are light brown and the seeds emit a toasted aroma.

Mix the sea salt and the toasted cumin in a mortar and grind them with a pestle. Peel the eggs and put them in a bowl. Toss with the salt and cumin mixture and serve.

Good for A, B, and C dieters.

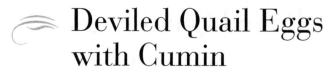

Deviled Quail Eggs with Cumin

SERVES 12.

Prepare the eggs and cumin seeds as in the previous recipe. Mix the cumin into the standard maconnaise recipe (see page 73), and set aside. Peel the eggs, cut them gently in half, remove the yolks, and place the yolks in a bowl. Leave the whites on a serving tray. Mash the yolks well, then mix the maconnaise/cumin mixture into them. Spoon this mixture into the halved egg whites and place back the whites back on the tray.

Good for A, B, and C dieters.

Garlic and Dill Feta Cheese Spread

MAKES 1 CUP.

This incredibly simple recipe was submitted by a patient from New Jersey who had never cooked before in her life. I challenged her to create a recipe for this book, and this is what she sent. It's simple, delicious, and incredibly easy to make.

8-ounce package cream cheese, softened
4-ounce package feta cheese, softened
¼ cup maconnaise (see recipe, page 73)
1 garlic clove, minced
1 tablespoon fresh dill, chopped
Salt
White pepper, freshly ground

Put all the ingredients into a food processor, and blend until the mixture is smooth. Cover and chill for 8 hours. Serve the spread with your favorite whole-grain chips or toast points.

Good for A, B, and C dieters.

Endive with Spanish Blue Cheese

SERVES 6.

Spanish blue cheese comes from the Picos de Europa mountains, located in Asturias in northern Spain. It is made from a blend of cow's and goat's milk and is matured in mountain caves for about three months. It has a strong smell and a smooth, creamy texture. It's a perfect accompaniment to the lemony endive. If you can't find Valdeon, cabrales, or tresviso, Roquefort is a good substitute.

12 white endives
4 ounces Spanish blue cheese
1 ounce cream cheese
2 tablespoons heavy cream
White pepper, freshly ground
Pinch nutmeg, freshly grated
Parsley, freshly chopped

Cut the rough end off the endives, about an eighth of an inch from the tip. Take off the large outer leaves and place them in a large bowl with enough ice and water to cover. This will make them nice and crisp. While they are soaking, make the cheese sauce.

In a large bowl, mix the cheeses and heavy cream well with a wooden spoon. Add the pepper and nutmeg and whisk the ingredients for about 2 minutes.

Drain the endive leaves, pat dry with a paper towel, and place 1 tablespoon of the cheese mixture in each endive leaf. Top with freshly chopped parsley.

Good for A, B, and C dieters.

Red Pepper Soup

This recipe was sent to me by one of my patients who lives in Boston. The consummate hostess, she was nervous about starting a new lifestyle program and was upset that her life might have to change. She was especially concerned about what this change could mean to her dinner parties. Needless to say, her chef has come up with many recipes. This is a simple yet elegant one that is perfect for entertaining, especially if it's served in demitasse cups. I have varied this recipe by using orange or yellow bell peppers, depending on the seasonality and the freshness of the supply, and each time, it comes out divine.

2 tablespoons macadamia nut oil
3¼ cups onions, sliced
3 cloves garlic, crushed
¼ cup dry white wine
12 large red bell peppers, cut into 1-inch pieces
2 cups chicken stock
½ jalapeño, seeded and sliced into cubes
2 tablespoons fresh thyme
2 tablespoons fresh chives
½ teaspoon fresh basil, chopped
½ teaspoon red pepper flakes

Put the oil in a large stockpot over medium-high heat. Add the onions, and sauté until they start to sweat, about 5 minutes. Add the garlic and cook for 1 more minute. Add the wine and cook it down almost completely. Add the bell peppers, stock, jalapeño, and all the herbs and additional spice. Cover and simmer until the peppers are tender, about 30 minutes. Pour the mixture into a food processor or blender, but don't adjust the seasonings yet—allow the heat of the jalapeño to come through.

Cover and chill the soup overnight or up to 2 days, or freeze portions to serve whenever you need a little something to spice up your dinner party. This soup can also be served warm. Either way, pour it into small champagne flutes and top with a dollop of sour cream or crème fraîche.

Good for A, B, and C dieters.

Baked Brie

SERVES 8–10.

This is a variation of another dish that was brought to my home one evening by a dear friend from Amagansett. On winter evenings, when no one wants to leave the house, we often have potluck dinners. People are always afraid to come to my house when I'm the host because they fear they will make something I don't approve of. That has almost never happened because eating the Hamptons Diet way allows for an incredibly varied diet.

8-inch round Brie cheese
2 fresh peaches, peeled
⅔ cup Pesto (recipe follows)
⅔ cup almonds, sliced

Preheat the oven to 325°F.

Place the cheese in a baking dish. Chop the peaches and lay them on top of the cheese. Spoon on the pesto and sprinkle with the almonds. Bake at 325°F for 15 minutes.

Pesto

2 cups fresh basil leaves
½ cup macadamia nut oil
3 cloves garlic, peeled and minced
3 tablespoons pine nuts
1 teaspoon salt
¼ teaspoon white pepper, freshly ground
¾ cup Parmesan cheese, grated

Put the basil leaves, olive oil, garlic cloves, pine nuts, salt, and pepper into a blender or food processor and blend on high, pushing the ingredients down occasionally until they are finely chopped. Remove to a bowl and add the grated cheese. To bring the pesto to a salad dressing consistency, add a tablespoon or two of hot water.

Good for A, B, and C dieters.

Shrimp-Stuffed Mushrooms

What dinner party or afternoon gathering would be complete without the wonderful stuffed mushroom? Sandra N. sent us this mushroom recipe, which is bound to please and excite your guests.

12 large fresh mushrooms, about 1 pound
Macadamia nut oil in a spray bottle
8 shrimp, cooked and chopped
¼ cup chicken broth
¼ teaspoon salt
¼ teaspoon cayenne pepper, ground
2 tablespoons Parmesan cheese, grated

Preheat oven to 375°F.

Remove the stems from the mushrooms and chop them. Spray the mushroom caps with macadamia nut oil. Stir together the stems, shrimp, and the remaining ingredients except the Parmesan cheese. Spoon evenly into the mushroom caps, then sprinkle the caps with the Parmesan cheese. Place the mushrooms on a lightly greased baking sheet and bake for 20 minutes.

Good for A, B, and C dieters.

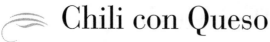

Chili con Queso

MAKES 6 CUPS.

This recipe was provided by my former house cleaner in Dallas. She loved to make all sorts of Mexican dishes for me, and this was one of my favorites. I served it to guests all the time, and they thought it was something out of this world.

1 pound hot pork sausage, ground
1 pound jalapeño jack cheese, cut into cubes
1 pound sharp cheddar cheese, cut into cubes
1 jar spicy salsa

In a large skillet, brown the sausage, stirring until it crumbles and is no longer pink; rinse, drain, and set aside. In a 2½-quart slow cooker, add the sausage and the remaining ingredients. Cover and cook the chili on low for 2 hours or until the cheese melts.

Good for A, B, and C dieters.

Marinated Goat Cheese with Olives and Whole Garlic

SERVES 12.

This combination is pure Mediterranean. Jeff discovered this dish during a trip to France with his brother. Jeff was living on the Costa Brava, one hour north of Barcelona, and they rented a car and drove through the Pyrenees up into France. They stopped for lunch at a little outdoor café, and right after they sat down, the owners brought this wonderful dish to their table.

12 8-ounce fresh goat cheese rounds
12 cloves of garlic
2 cups macadamia nut oil
¾ cup Niçoise olives
1 teaspoon salt
1 teaspoon black pepper, freshly ground
1 teaspoon red pepper flakes
1 tablespoon fresh rosemary
3 bay leaves

Try to find firm 8-ounce goat cheese rounds, small enough to marinate whole. Peel the garlic and place in a small sauté pan. Cover with macadamia nut oil and cook over very low heat until the garlic is tender but firm, about 10 minutes. Drain, reserving the oil. Let the garlic cool to room temperature.

Place the cheese in a jar large enough to hold it. Add the garlic, olives, salt, black pepper, red pepper flakes, rosemary, and bay leaves. Cover the cheese with the garlic-infused macadamia nut oil and the rest of the plain macadamia nut oil, making sure to completely cover the cheese. Cover the jar and marinate the cheese in a cool place for at least 24 hours.

Serve it with your favorite crisp fresh vegetables.

Good for A, B, and C dieters.

Roasted Almonds with Paprika

SERVES 6–8.

Jeff's first tapas experience was in Granada, where he drank sherry and was given his first little bites to eat. One of the dishes he fondly remembers was almonds with paprika because they went so well with the dry sherry. Both the almonds and the sherry come from just outside of Granada. There is no sherry in this recipe, but on a cold winter's night, this would make an ideal appetizer served with sherry as an aperitif as the guests arrive.

10 ounces whole blanched almonds
1 tablespoon macadamia nut oil
1 teaspoon smoked Spanish paprika
1¼ teaspoons fine sea salt

Preheat the oven to 450°F.

Place the almonds on a baking tray and dry roast them in the oven for about 5 to 8 minutes or until golden brown. Remove from the oven and stir in the macadamia nut oil, paprika, and salt. Return the tray to the oven for about 5 minutes. Remove from the oven and let cool for 15 minutes before serving.

Good for A, B, and C dieters.

Spicy Almonds

This is another dish that can be created with almost any nut you prefer. A nice variation is to use mixed fresh nuts. I recommend almonds, walnuts, or macadamia nuts since they are the heart-healthiest, but feel free to use whichever nuts you like. Use one type of nut on one occasion and another for a different meal if you wish.

1 pound whole blanched almonds
1 tablespoon smoked Spanish paprika
1 teaspoon cayenne pepper
1 tablespoon salt
1 tablespoon macadamia nut oil

Preheat the oven to 350°F.

Spread out the almonds on a cookie sheet and place in the oven. Bake for about 6 to 7 minutes or until lightly brown and the almonds start to make a popping noise. While the almonds are toasting, mix the spices and salt in a large bowl. Remove the almonds from the oven and, while they're still hot, put them in the bowl with the spices. Add the oil and mix well to coat the almonds evenly. Return the almonds to the cookie sheet to cool. Check the salt to taste and add more if necessary. Store the almonds in an airtight container. These go great with olives.

Good for A, B, and C dieters.

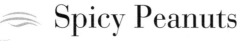

Spicy Peanuts

SERVES 10–12.

If you like things really spicy hot, then these spicy peanuts are just the snack for you! This is another recipe that can be made ahead of time and then parceled into 1-ounce packages to ensure that you don't overeat them. They can easily be taken to school or work or sent to a sleepover. If these peanuts are too hot, simply eliminate the cayenne pepper. Since most people will eat peanuts, that is the nut we used in this recipe. Any nut will do, however, and, given the number of children with peanut allergies, you may want to stick with almonds, cashews, or walnuts.

1 cup raw peanuts
1 teaspoon salt
¼ teaspoon chili powder
¼ teaspoon sweet paprika
¼ teaspoon cayenne pepper
1 tablespoon macadamia nut oil

Preheat the oven to 325°F.

Combine all the ingredients in a large bowl and mix well. Spread out the peanuts on a cookie sheet and bake 5 to 10 minutes, stirring once, until they're nicely toasted.

Good for A, B, and C dieters.

Marinated Olives

It's fun to pick and choose your own olives for this dish, but unless you live in California, that's probably not going to happen. It's best to use olives with the pits still inside them, but pitted olives work almost as well. Look for a variety of tastes, colors, and textures. Some kinds of olives to consider are kalamata, Niçoise, arbequina, manzanilla, petit lucques, or douces.

1 pound mixed olives in brine
1 small Spanish onion
1 red onion
1 red bell pepper
1 green bell pepper
1 garlic clove, minced
1 lemon, quartered
1 tablespoon whole black peppercorns
1 teaspoon red pepper flakes
1 tablespoon parsley, chopped
1 tablespoon fresh thyme, chopped
1 tablespoon fresh rosemary, chopped
¾ cup extra-virgin olive oil

Drain the olives from their brine, rinse briefly under cold water, and place in a large bowl. Dice the Spanish and red onions and red and green bell peppers. Place in the bowl with the olives. Add the remaining ingredients. Mix well and cover the bowl with plastic wrap. Let marinate for 24 hours before serving.

Good for A, B, and C dieters.

Parmesan Crackers

MAKES 40 CRACKERS.

The next two recipes are for those of you who can't live without breadlike prod-ucts. I personally recommend that you try to find a whole-grain cracker or something like that, or do what I do and just eat the dip or the spread off the cracker without actually putting it in your mouth. Because not everyone has as much willpower as I do, I thought I would add a few recipes that require pro-tein powders and that hark back to my low-carbohydrate roots. So, for anyone who still likes to count carbohydrates, these two recipes are for you. Of course, they are low glycemic. I originally devised these recipes for a supper party I was having with some powerful television producers. They were very skeptical of any-thing low carbohydrate at that time, and I wanted to prove to them that they would never be able to tell the difference. To this day, they think they ate store-bought crackers.

1 cup whey protein powder
1 teaspoon baking powder
½ teaspoon sea salt
1 egg
¼ cup water
½ cup Parmesan cheese, grated
2 tablespoons butter, melted, or macadamia nut oil

Preheat the oven to 325°F.

Mix the whey powder, baking powder, salt, egg, water, and grated cheese together in a bowl.

Line a cookie sheet with parchment paper and grease the paper with melted butter or macadamia nut oil. Drop the batter by teaspoonfuls onto the paper, keeping them three inches apart.

Bake the crackers for 10 to 12 minutes, until golden, rotating the pan 180° halfway through the cooking time. Remove to a cooling rack.

Good for A, B, and C dieters. A: 3 crackers; B: 6 crackers; C: 8 crackers.

Cheddar Crackers

Follow the Parmesan Crackers recipe, replacing the Parmesan cheese with shredded cheddar cheese and adding 3 tablespoons of dried parsley flakes.

Swiss Crackers

Follow the Parmesan Crackers recipe, replacing the Parmesan cheese with shredded Swiss cheese and adding 3 tablespoons of dried dill weed.

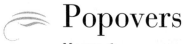

Popovers

Makes 6.

You will need a popover pan with six sections or a heavy muffin pan, not aluminum, or small custard cups on a cookie sheet.

½ cup unflavored whey protein
2 tablespoons butter, melted
½ cup heavy cream
¾ cup water
2 eggs
¼ teaspoon sea salt
2 tablespoons macadamia nut oil

Preheat the oven to 425°F.

Grease the popover cups with softened butter. Heat them in the preheated oven for 10 minutes. Whisk together the whey protein, melted butter, cream, water, eggs, and sea salt.

Place 1 teaspoon of oil in each cup, and immediately pour the batter evenly into the hot cups until each one is two-thirds full.

Bake at 425°F for 15 minutes. Reduce the heat to 325°F, and continue baking for another 12 minutes.

Serve the popovers with butter or flavored butter or remove the tops and fill them with your favorite salad, cheese, or meat.

For variety, add 1 tablespoon of dried parsley flakes or dill weed (or whatever herbs or spices you fancy) to the batter before cooking.

Good for A, B, and C dieters.

Roasted Asparagus with Mountain Ham

SERVES 8–12.

The Italians have prosciutto, the Spanish have serrano, and Americans have country ham. All are aged from several months to several years. You can use any of them for this recipe, but just make sure that the one you buy is very finely sliced.

¼ cup macadamia nut oil
12 slices serrano ham or prosciutto
24 medium asparagus spears
White pepper, freshly ground

Preheat the oven to 400°F.

Put half the oil in a roasting pan that will hold the asparagus spears in a single layer and swirl the pan around so the oil covers the bottom. Cut each slice of ham in half lengthwise. Trim the ends of the asparagus spears, then wrap a slice of ham around the stem end of each spear. Place the wrapped spears in the prepared roasting pan and lightly brush the ham and asparagus with the remaining oil. Season the spears with pepper.

Roast the asparagus spears in the oven for 10 minutes, depending on the thickness of the asparagus, or until tender but still firm. Do not overcook the asparagus—it's important that the spears stay firm. Serve piping hot.

Good for A, B, and C dieters.

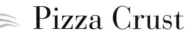

Pizza Crust

SERVES 8.

Here is the recipe every mother and child have been waiting for. As with most foods, it's possible to make pizza crust healthier simply by switching some of the ingredients. Jeff chose to make this particular recipe using soy flour; however, you can use almost any whole-grain flour you desire. This recipe is great with whole wheat flour; my favorite is with spelt flour. It's just a simple recipe. What's most important with pizza is what's on top of the crust, and that is limited only by your budget and imagination.

4 eggs
1 cup heavy cream
½ cup seltzer water
1½ teaspoons salt
2 cups soy flour
Macadamia nut oil

Preheat the oven to 350°F.

In a mixing bowl, beat the eggs until the yolks and whites are combined. Pour in the cream and seltzer water. Add the salt and stir in the soy flour. The mixture will be slightly liquid.

Lightly oil 3 individual-size pizza pans (about 9 inches). Spread the batter thinly on the pans.

Bake until slightly browned and partially cooked through, about 7 minutes. Add your favorite toppings and return the pans to the oven. These crusts can even be made far ahead of time and frozen, so you can always have a pizza handy when the kids or your husband is clamoring for one.

Good for B and C dieters.

Pizza Sauce

8-ounce can stewed tomatoes
1 teaspoon dried oregano
Salt
Black pepper, freshly ground
2 tablespoons macadamia nut oil

In a small saucepan, add all the ingredients and bring to a simmer for 15 minutes. Pass the sauce through a ricer or put it in a blender on low speed for just a few seconds until it's well combined. Spread the sauce on the crust, add your favorite toppings, and bake the pizza.

Good for B and C dieters.

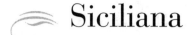

Siciliana

MAKES ENOUGH FOR 1 PIZZA.

Pizza Crust (see recipe, page 230)
Pizza Sauce (see recipe, page 231)
1 ripe tomato, sliced
1 cup mozzarella, shredded
½ cup fresh basil, chopped

Top the pizza crust with the pizza sauce.

Add slices of fresh tomato and freshly grated mozzarella. Place the pizza in a preheated oven of 350°F for 6 to 7 minutes. Remove from the oven and top with chopped fresh basil.

Good for B and C dieters.

Ham and Cheese Pizza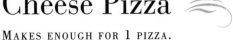

MAKES ENOUGH FOR 1 PIZZA.

Pizza Crust (see recipe, page 230)
Pizza Sauce (see recipe, page 231)
4 ounces ham (any kind will do in this recipe—in fact,
    any meat can be substituted, including meatballs,
    sausage, and pepperoni, all nitrite-free)
½ cup mozzarella, shredded
½ cup Monterey Jack cheese, shredded

Top the pizza crust with the pizza sauce, then add slices of ham, and top with
your favorite cheese. (As with the meat, the cheeses suggested in the recipe are
only two examples of the types you can use.) Place the pizza in a preheated
350°F oven for 6 to 7 minutes. Remove from the oven, allow to cool for 3 minutes, slice, and serve.

Good for B and C dieters.

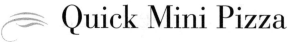

Quick Mini Pizza

SERVES 1.

I don't know a finicky person in the world who doesn't like pizza. Here is an idea to make a quick pizza snack. The base is a whole-grain muffin and tomato sauce. Aside from those two ingredients, you can add whatever you want as a topping as long as it stays within the guidelines of the health pyramids. This dish is near and dear to my heart because my mother always made it for me.

2 tablespoons tomato sauce, nonsugar (preferably organic;
   canned is fine)
½ whole-grain English muffin
1 tablespoon fresh basil, chopped
2 tablespoons mozzarella cheese, grated
Pepperoni, nitrate-free

Preheat the broiler.

Spread the tomato sauce evenly over the English muffin. Sprinkle with the fresh basil and mozzarella, then top with the pepperoni. Broil until the cheese is brown and the sauce is hot. Serve immediately.

Good for A, B, and C dieters.

Stuffed Pimientos

SERVES 12.

If you can find pimientos de piquillo from Spain, get some. They are smoked, sweet, and spicy red peppers. Make sure they are whole and not sliced. If you can't find them, instead look for a jar of peppadew peppers from South Africa.

2 cups ricotta cheese
1 tablespoon macadamia nut oil
1 tablespoon lemon juice
1 garlic clove, minced
½ cup fresh flat-leaf parsley, chopped
1 tablespoon fresh mint, chopped
1 tablespoon fresh thyme, chopped
1 tablespoon fresh chives, chopped, plus more for garnish
Salt
White pepper, freshly ground
2 6-ounce bottles or cans of pimientos de piquillo

For the cheese filling, put all the ingredients except for the peppers into a large glass bowl and mix well with a large wooden spoon. Using a teaspoon, stuff each pepper with the cheese filling. Refrigerate the stuffed peppers for about 2 hours until they're firm.

To serve the peppers, arrange them on a serving plate, and, if necessary, wipe them with a paper towel to remove any of the filling that has spread over the skins. Garnish with chopped chives.

Good for A, B, and C dieters.

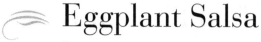

Eggplant Salsa

SERVES 6–8.

1 large or 2 medium eggplants
1 jalapeño pepper
½ teaspoon salt, plus extra to taste
¼ cup macadamia nut oil
3 large garlic cloves, minced

Place the eggplants and the jalapeño pepper on a baking sheet in a preheated 400°F oven. Bake for 40 minutes or until the eggplant is soft to the touch through an oven mitt. Remove from the oven and let cool to room temperature. Remove the ends and skin from the eggplant and mash it very well in a mixing bowl. Mince the jalapeño and add it to the eggplant. Add the salt. Mince the garlic and mix it into the eggplant mixture. Add the macadamia nut oil and thoroughly mix all the ingredients. Chill.

When you are ready to serve it, taste the salsa to see if it needs a bit more salt. This is great as a fresh veggie dip, or put a dollop on a slice of fresh buffalo mozzarella and serve it as an appetizer.

Good for A, B, and C dieters.

Crabmeat Dip

This is Jeff's girlfriend's recipe, which she invented three summers ago. At every party she has ever taken the dish to, someone has asked for the recipe. Jeff did the same thing after he tried it the first time. Here is a tip: the better the crabmeat, the better the dip.

8-ounce package cream cheese
½ cup maconnaise (see recipe, page 73)
Juice of 1 lemon, freshly squeezed
¼ teaspoon Tabasco sauce
½ teaspoon red pepper flakes
Salt
Black pepper, freshly ground
¼ red bell pepper, chopped
¼ green bell pepper, chopped
2 tablespoons red onion, chopped and rinsed
2 tablespoons green onion, chopped
3 7-ounce cans crabmeat, drained

Soften the cream cheese in a large bowl by allowing it to sit at room temperature for 1 hour. Using a fork or hand mixer, combine the cheese with the maconnaise, lemon juice, Tabasco, red pepper flakes, salt, and black pepper. Then add the rest of the ingredients and mix well. Adjust the seasoning and refrigerate the dip for at least 2 hours. Recheck the seasoning one more time before serving the dip.

Good for A, B, and C dieters.

Deviled Eggs with Crabmeat

SERVES 12.

This recipe is a simple variation on the previous one. Cooking healthy or just eating in a healthy way is really easy! If I could convince Chef Jeff, I ought to be able to convince you.

10 eggs
¼ cup maconnaise (see recipe, page 73)
2 tablespoons celery, minced
1 tablespoon parsley, chopped
3 teaspoons Dijon mustard
4 drops Worcestershire sauce
2 drops Tabasco sauce
Salt
Black pepper, freshly ground
7-ounce can crabmeat, drained
Paprika

Place the eggs in 2 quarts of salted cold water. Bring the water to a boil and boil the eggs for 10 minutes. Drain and immediately place the eggs in about 2 quarts of ice water for 10 minutes. This will keep the yolks from turning gray instead of staying a bright yellow. Peel the eggs and cut them in half lengthwise. Remove the yolks to a large bowl and set aside the egg whites. Mash the yolks with a fork. In the same bowl as the yolks, add all the ingredients except the crabmeat and the paprika and mix well. Add the crabmeat and mix it through completely. Fill the egg whites with the yolk mixture and sprinkle with paprika. Cover and refrigerate for 1 hour before serving.

Good for A, B, and C dieters.

Figs Wrapped in Prosciutto

SERVING SIZE = 1 FIG.

10 thin slices prosciutto
20 black mission figs

Preheat the oven to 400°F.

Cut each piece of prosciutto in half lengthwise. Wrap 1 piece of prosciutto around each fig. Place each wrapped fig on a cookie sheet and put the cookie sheet in the oven for 5 minutes. Serve immediately.

Good for B and C dieters.

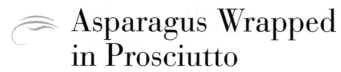

Asparagus Wrapped in Prosciutto

SERVES 10.

10 thin slices prosciutto
20 medium asparagus stalks

Preheat the oven to 400°F.

Cut each piece of prosciutto in half lengthwise. Bring 2 quarts of salted water to a rapid boil. Drop in the asparagus stalks for 30 seconds, then drain them. Run cold water over the asparagus until it's no longer hot. Pat the asparagus dry with a paper towel. Wrap each stalk of asparagus with prosciutto. Place all the asparagus stalks on a cookie sheet and bake for 5 minutes. Serve immediately.

Good for A, B, and C dieters.

Melon with Prosciutto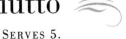

SERVES 5.

10 thin slices prosciutto
1 cantaloupe

Cut each piece of prosciutto in half lengthwise. Cut the cantaloupe in half. Remove the seeds and cut off the rough outer skin. Cut the cantaloupe into 20 bite-size pieces. Using toothpicks, fold the prosciutto over 3 times, then stick a toothpick through it, then into a melon piece. Repeat with all of the prosciutto and cantaloupe. Put all of the pieces on a plate, and refrigerate until you're ready to serve them.

Good for A, B, and C dieters.

Prosciutto and Chèvre Roll-Ups

SERVES 12.

This recipe can actually be made with any soft cheese, including standard American cream cheese. Just note that because prosciutto has such a strong and salty flavor, you need a cheese that can stand up to the saltiness.

4 ounces cream cheese
4 ounces soft goat cheese
1 tablespoon fresh thyme, chopped
1 tablespoon fresh parsley, chopped
1 tablespoon fresh chives, chopped
½ cup pine nuts, toasted
Kosher salt
White pepper, freshly ground
10 pieces of prosciutto, thinly sliced
2 cups arugula

With a wooden spoon stir together the first eight ingredients in a large bowl. Lay the prosciutto on a baking sheet or large sheet of aluminum foil. Spread about 2 tablespoons of the cheese mixture over each prosciutto slice. Top each with some arugula.

Roll up each slice from the short side and cut into half-inch-thick slices. Serve immediately or cover and chill up to 4 hours.

Good for A, B, and C dieters.

Italian Celery Bites

This is a popular dish served toward the end of summer in Tuscany. The pine nuts add that first taste of fall.

8 ounces cream cheese
4 ounces Parmesan, grated
¼ cup pine nuts, toasted
¼ cup sundried tomatoes, chopped
1 teaspoon oregano, dried (or freshly chopped from your herb garden, if possible)
Salt
Black pepper, freshly ground
10 celery stalks, trimmed

Mix all the ingredients in a large bowl. If you're not serving the dish immediately, don't include the pine nuts in this step. Set them aside. Sprinkle the pine nuts on top of each stalk just prior to serving.

Remove the tops and the wide base from the celery. Using a vegetable peeler, remove two thin strips from the rounded side of the celery, creating a flat surface so the celery will lie flat. Stuff each stalk with the cheese filling and serve.

Good for A, B, and C dieters.

Cucumber and Feta Bites

SERVES 10–12.

This is a mini version of a traditional Greek salad. I have served this many times, and despite its simplicity, it never fails to impress. This is a great dish for vegetarians (but not vegans, of course) and makes a great salad course when you really don't want to add a regular salad to the menu.

1 cup feta cheese, crumbled
½ cup sour cream
3 tablespoons fresh parsley, chopped
2 tablespoons fresh mint, chopped
3 tablespoons sundried tomatoes, chopped
1 clove garlic, chopped
Salt
Black pepper, freshly ground
2 medium cucumbers
¼ cup fresh basil, chopped
¼ cup kalamata olives, pitted and chopped

In a large bowl, mix the first eight ingredients. Cover and chill for at least 2 hours.

Using a sharp knife, trim the ends from the cucumber. Slice the cucumber into quarter-inch-thick slices. Spoon about 1 teaspoon of the cheese mixture onto each cucumber slice. Arrange the cucumber slices on a serving platter.

In a small bowl, combine the basil and the olives. Spoon some of the mixture over each cucumber slice. Serve immediately.

Good for A, B, and C dieters.

Indian Puffed Quinoa

SERVES 10–12.

Indian cuisine is known for its excellent curry dishes. This Indian quinoa shines when you use a high-quality curry. It's actually served just like popcorn would be, and you could also use puffed brown rice or a puffed whole wheat pasta kernel to make this dish. Your guests will never know it isn't popcorn.

½ teaspoon Madras curry
¼ teaspoon ground turmeric
Pinch cinnamon
Pinch nutmeg
Pinch cayenne pepper
Salt
Black pepper, freshly ground
Puffed quinoa
Macadamia nut oil in a spray bottle

Mix the first seven ingredients in a large bowl. Lay out the quinoa on a cookie sheet and spray it lightly with macadamia nut oil. Put the quinoa in the bowl with the spices, mix well, and serve.

Good for B and C dieters.

8

Hamptons Diet Desserts

A cookbook wouldn't be complete without a chapter dedicated to most Americans' favorite part of the meal—the sweet. In real life, I advocate to my patients that a small piece of fruit is the best and healthiest dessert—it has great antioxidants and phytonutrients and is low calorie to boot. In this chapter, however, I wanted to show the world that it's possible to make indulgent desserts that aren't hazardous to your health. Please consider, though, that if you want to be thin and healthy for the long haul, dessert just won't be a big part of your life.

A Word on Sweeteners

Sugar won't be used in any of these dessert recipes. Recently, a plethora of new things to satisfy your sweet tooth have hit the market, many of which are just as dangerous as sugar. There are too many for me to write about here, but I'll mention some of the ones you'll see in this chapter and some of the ones you should simply avoid.

Healthy Sweeteners

+ Lo-Han fruit is my favorite sweetener, and I think it would be more popular if it weren't so expensive. Made from a fruit grown in Japan, it's noncaloric and completely natural. The reason it's my favorite is that it works like sugar and it looks like brown sugar, and there is almost no conversion needed for your favorite recipes. It creates texture, helps to bind foods, caramelizes, and does all the yummy things we expect from sugar.

+ Stevia is my second-favorite sweetener. It's derived from a plant that grows wild in the tropical rain forest, and it is completely non-nutritive (meaning it doesn't add calories) and completely natural. It is 600 times sweeter than sugar, so it can be a little difficult to use. Something that sweet is bitter when too much is used, and finding the right amount is tricky; however, it can be done. Stevia does not caramelize and will not add texture and mouth feel to your dishes, but it will sweeten them quite safely and satisfyingly.

+ Xylitol has a glycemic index of only 7, which is very low. Although it falls into the family of sugar alcohols, it is chemically different. Xylitol is a natural product that regularly occurs in the glucose metabolism of humans, other animals, and some plants. Unlike other alternative sweeteners, Xylitol can be digested by enzymes in our bodies, and, therefore, gastric upset is usually not a problem. If you do have a problem, after three days, your body should adjust.

+ Agave fruit concentrate is a sweetener that you'll see with increasing frequency. It's made from the agave fruit and is low glycemic. It's still a sugar and acts like that in the body, and calories must be taken into consideration, but it's absorbed quite slowly, so for people following a low-GI diet, it's an ideal sweetener.

+ Saccharin was taken off the list of known carcinogens and probably should not have been put there in the first place. It is a safe sweetener and is something I often use in dessert recipes. The problem is that it cannot be used to thicken or bind foods together. If you use this as a sweetener, you will always have to use more eggs. Saccharin can be used for glazes, as it will caramelize at high heat.

The "Jury's Still Out" Sweeteners

+ Splenda is also known as sucralose and has become extremely popular recently. It is found in many mainstream diet products. Although there are some recipes in this chapter that call for its use, the jury is still out on the safety of this sweetener. I personally never use it, but due to its cooking characteristics, chefs love to use it. It does exactly what sugar does, in terms of binding foods and giving them the appropriate mouth feel. It is, however, chlorinated sugar; chlorine is a known carcinogen, and I'm uncomfortable recommending it until we see what happens now that it is fully introduced into the mass market.

+ Tagatose is a new one on the market and is backed by a big food manufacturing company, so be prepared to see this one everywhere soon. As it is brand new, I'm unsure of its side effects. I am of the mind that if it's man-made and new, I avoid it for five years until I see what it is doing to others.

+ Maltitol, sorbitol, and erythritol were and still are found in products labeled "low carb" or "for diabetics." They do not raise blood sugar as much as regular sugar does, but they do add calories, and their carbohydrate content must be counted into the mix. Many people who start to consume products that contain these sweeteners fail to lose weight. The laxative effects can also be quite pronounced.

Sweeteners to Avoid

+ Nutrasweet is the most common artificial sweetener you will see, next to Splenda. This is the most harmful one to date. Although it's not widely recognized as a neurotoxin, there are thousands of reported cases throughout the world of people who have experienced brain injuries from overconsumption of this sweetener. At the very least, do me one favor and please don't serve it to anyone under the age of eighteen.

✦ Brown rice syrup is commonly found in "no sugar added" products and is also in rice milk. It is very sweet, with a high glycemic index. Please avoid it.

✦ Barley malt should be avoided for the same reason as brown rice syrup.

Please note that with these dessert recipes, the number of servings is approximate. I like to make more than one dessert so that my guests can have a taste of several different things, but you may have time to make only one dessert. Be aware of this when you check the numbers of servings for the recipes in this section.

Chilled Almond Soup with Oven-Roasted Figs and Coconut Mascarpone

SERVES 8.

Almonds have been used in Spain since the Moors introduced them in the eighth century. Since then, the Spanish have been very creative in their use of this versatile nut. Today you can find almonds in every aspect of Spanish cooking, from sauces to soups, from tapas to stews, and from puddings to cakes. The fruit is harvested in August and September along the Mediterranean coast.

3 cups raw almonds, soaked for 10 to 12 hours in bottled water,
    rinsed, and drained
6 cups bottled water
1 can unsweetened coconut milk
1 teaspoon stevia
½ cup heavy cream
1 cup mascarpone cheese
8 black mission figs (or, alternately, peaches)

In a blender, combine the almonds and the 6 cups bottled water and blend until creamy. Pour the mixture into a sieve lined with cheesecloth. Let it drain for about an hour, then push out as much of the milk as you can, using the back of a ladle. Put the almond milk in a covered container and refrigerate for up to 3 days. Makes 4 cups.

Put the coconut milk in a medium saucepan over medium-low heat. Bring to a simmer and add the stevia, stirring occasionally. Reduce the liquid by half. Transfer it to a glass bowl and refrigerate for about 1 hour, until well chilled.

With a hand mixer, whip the heavy cream in a chilled stainless steel bowl until stiff. Fold the mascarpone into the cream. Whisk the mixture again until stiff. Fold in the reduced coconut milk. Refrigerate the mixture until it's needed.

Preheat the broiler.

Chilled Almond Soup with Oven-Roasted Figs and Coconut Mascarpone (*continued*)

Cut the figs in half lengthwise. Place the figs cut-side down on a baking sheet. Put the baking sheet in the oven on the top rack or 6 inches from the broiler. Broil for 3 to 4 minutes or until lightly browned and caramelized.

To plate, pour ½ cup of almond milk into each bowl. Place 1 heaping tablespoon of the mascarpone mixture in the middle of the almond milk. Place 2 warm fig halves on top of the mascarpone and serve.

Good for B and C dieters.

Custard with Cherries

SERVES 8.

Eggs, milk, and sugar were the basis of most desserts during medieval times in Europe. From this simple combination came many classics that are commonly found throughout the world today, including custard. We know better now and can make this healthier by replacing the sugar. This recipe is a great base for many desserts because you can change the fruit depending on the season.

3 cups heavy cream
Zest of 1 lemon
1 teaspoon vanilla extract
4 egg yolks
2 eggs
1 teaspoon lo-han
1 pound fresh cherries

Put the heavy cream, lemon zest, and vanilla in a saucepan over medium heat. Bring to a simmer, remove from the heat, and let sit for 10 minutes. In a large bowl, add the yolks, eggs, and lo-han. Mix well. Pour the cream mixture back into the saucepan and place it over very low heat, stirring constantly for 15 to 20 minutes, until thick. Remove the pan from the heat and strain the liquid into a metal bowl. Place this bowl over a bowl containing ice water, to chill. If the custard gets lumpy while you are cooking it, place the pan in the ice water and whisk the custard well. Spoon the custard into bowls and refrigerate for about 1 hour until well chilled.

Cut the cherries in half and remove the pits. Place four cherry halves on top of the chilled custard and serve.

Good for A, B, and C dieters.

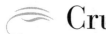

Crunchy Pear Boat

SERVES 1.

You will find plenty of energy and good nutrition in these little boats. They are an elegant dessert for a dinner party and are simple enough to send to school or make after a long, hard day at the office. The other great thing about this recipe is that you can use any fruit that's in season, fresh, or local that day at the market. You can also vary this recipe by changing the nut butters or mixing two different types in the same boat.

1 ripe pear
2 tablespoons peanut butter, natural, sugar-free
2 tablespoons granola, sugar-free, either store bought
   or you can use the recipe on page 41
Chocolate Whipped Cream for garnish (optional) (see recipe, page 255)

Wash and dry the pear. Cut it in half lengthwise and remove the seeds. Place the pear halves in a sundae dish and spread the nut butter into the cored area of the fruit and around the edges. Sprinkle granola on top. To make this extra special, you can top it with Chocolate Whipped Cream.

Chocolate Whipped Cream

MAKES 1 CUP.

1 cup heavy cream
1 teaspoon lo-han, or stevia to taste (optional)
1 tablespoon unsweetened cocoa

Pour the cream into a cold stainless steel bowl—I put mine in the freezer for up to 1 hour before using it—and, with an electric mixer set on the highest speed, whip the cream until just before it starts to form peaks. Add the sweetener, if you would like, at this point and continue to whip the cream. Add the unsweetened cocoa and whip until stiff peaks form. This is a great addition to the Pear Boat recipe.

Good for A, B, and C dieters.

Apricot Pistachio Balls

SERVING SIZE—1 BALL.

This and the following recipe came from a Moroccan whom Jeff met in Madrid. For the apricot balls, use the natural tart variety of dried apricots, not the sweetened or honeyed ones; they should be soft. Both the Apricot Pistachio Balls and the Date Walnut Balls keep for several weeks.

1 pound dried apricots
1 cup pistachios, shelled, finely chopped
1 tablespoon macadamia nut oil (optional)

Do not soak or wash the apricots, or you will produce a cream. Put the dried apricots in a food processor and blend them to a smooth paste, adding a teaspoon of water if needed. Wet your hands with water or put 1 tablespoon of macadamia nut oil on your hands so that the paste doesn't stick. Roll a teaspoon of the paste into a marble-sized ball with your greased hands. Continue until the paste is gone. Roll these balls in the chopped pistachios and serve.

Good for A, B, and C dieters.

Date Walnut Balls

1 pound dried pitted dates, soft and moist
1 pound walnuts, coarsely chopped

Blend the dates in a food processor and reduce to a paste. Add the walnuts and mix well. Shape into marble-sized balls and serve.

Good for A, B, and C dieters.

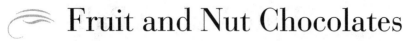

Fruit and Nut Chocolates

SERVING SIZE—1 BALL.

Jeff created these chocolate treats for a friend who has diabetes. They are great little sweet treats, with lots of flavor in a small package.

½ cup dried apricots
¼ cup dried figs
¼ cup almonds, sliced
¼ cup walnuts, chopped
¼ cup lemon juice, freshly squeezed
4 ounces bittersweet chocolate

Put the fruit and nuts into a food processor and chop until they're small. Add the lemon juice and chop again. Scrape the mixture into a bowl and taste it to see if more lemon juice is needed. Melt the chocolate in a heatproof bowl in the microwave for about 2 minutes or, preferably, over a double boiler, until it's just melted. Roll the fruit mixture into small balls. Using two forks, roll each ball in the melted chocolate. Place the balls on oiled foil to cool and set. If the chocolate gets too hard to work with, briefly reheat it.

Good for A, B, and C dieters.

Coconut Mousse

These are two things that can't be left out of a good cookbook: coconut, because of its great flavor, and mousse, because it's fun to learn the technique. Coconut also has great health properties because of the high levels of lauric acid found in its milk.

⅓ cup unsweetened coconut milk, divided
2 (¼-ounce) packages unflavored gelatin
2 cups heavy cream
4 egg whites
3 packets Splenda or 3 teaspoons lo-han
1 cup coconut, toasted, for garnish (optional) (recipe follows)

Place 4 tablespoons of the coconut milk into a small saucepan with the gelatin. Heat over low heat until the gelatin dissolves, stirring constantly, about 1 minute. Remove from the heat and set aside to cool.

With a hand blender in a chilled stainless steel bowl, whip the heavy cream to soft peaks and fold in the rest of the coconut milk.

In a separate bowl, whip the egg whites to soft peaks, slowly adding the Splenda or the lo-han toward the end of the process, creating a meringue.

Fold the gelatin mixture into the meringue, then fold in the whipped cream. Put the mousse in serving dishes or glasses and cover them with plastic wrap. Refrigerate for 3 to 4 hours or overnight. Before serving, sprinkle with toasted coconut, if you like.

Toasted Coconut Garnish

½ cup unsweetened coconut flakes
Macadamia nut oil in a spray bottle
⅛ cup lo-han

Toasted Coconut Garnish (*continued*)

To toast the coconut, simply place the unsweetened coconut flakes on a cookie sheet, spray with macadamia nut oil, and sprinkle with the lo-han. Toast in a preheated 350°F oven for about 4 to 6 minutes. Do not overcook. Allow the coconut to cool to room temperature before using. This garnish can be made ahead of time, and you can also make extra by doubling the recipe.

Good for A, B, and C dieters.

Macadamia Nut Ice Cream

MAKES 1½ PINTS.

This recipe and the following two were sent to me by a lovely woman in Dallas named Anne Strier. She was a chef for many years, and because of all her experience, she makes great food in a way that many cooks of today have completely forgotten. This dish is out of this world. Anne managed to make one of the world's most unhealthy foods (albeit my favorite food) into a very healthy treat. The basic formula has a creamy, nutty, unforgettable flavor.

½ cup macadamia nut oil
2 cups heavy cream
¾ cup sugar substitute of your choice
½ cup pasteurized egg whites
1 tablespoon vanilla extract

Whisk all the ingredients together in a bowl. Freeze the mixture in a shallow pan or ice cream maker until firm. Serve the ice cream plain or with crushed macadamia nuts, or you can spread it in a chilled crumb crust (recipe follows) and freeze until it's firm.

Chocolate Macadamia Nut Ice Cream

MAKES 1½ PINTS.

½ cup cocoa powder, unsweetened
½ cup macadamia nuts (or any nut of your choice), chopped, toasted

Combine the ingredients from the previous recipe as well as the cocoa powder and macadamia nuts and follow the preparation instructions from the previous recipe.

Good for A, B, and C dieters.

Macadamia Nut Crumb Crust

MAKES ONE 9-INCH PIE CRUST.

This crust goes perfectly with the Macadamia Nut Ice Cream to make an ice cream pie the kids will love. It's a great way to get in a lot of monounsaturated heart-healthy fat in a dessert setting.

This pie crust may also be used for a meringue-type pie or for any custard pies. Meringue is nothing more than egg whites, and custards are essentially just yolks and cream, so there are many variations to the following simple recipes. This is another example of the fine art of learning just a few tricks and all the variations—the Hamptons Diet cooking methodology.

1 cup macadamia nuts (or, alternatively, almonds), toasted
½ cup miller's bran
¼ cup lo-han or other sugar substitute
6 tablespoons macadamia nut oil

Preheat the oven to 350°F.

Put the nuts on a cookie sheet and toast for about 5 minutes or until just brown—do not overcook. Put the nuts, bran, sugar substitute, and oil into a food processor. Pulse until everything is crumbled together. Press this mixture into the bottom of a 9-inch pie pan and bake it for 10 to 12 minutes until lightly browned. Remove it from the oven, add your pie fillings, and bake according to the pie recipe's instructions. Or, you can premake a lot of these crusts, allow them to cool completely, and freeze them. This way, you are always prepared for guests or for when you need a sweet yet healthy treat.

Good for A, B, and C dieters.

Meringue Pie

MAKES A 9-INCH PIE FILLING.

This is a simple recipe that you can use over and over again in different settings. Once you've mastered the basic meringue, you can add unsweetened chocolate, fruit essences, and various extracts to get different taste sensations. This is not a traditional lemon meringue–type recipe, which is meringue over custard. I separate the two because the meringue is a low-calorie and lower-carbohydrate treat. The custard pies are a little heavier and somewhat more caloric.

2 egg whites
¼ teaspoon cream of tartar
3 tablespoons lo-han or Splenda (this recipe works best
   with these two sweeteners)
½ teaspoon vanilla extract
1 Macadamia Nut Crumb Crust (see recipe, page 262)

Preheat oven to 350°F.

   In a medium-sized mixing bowl, whip the egg whites until frothy. Add the cream of tartar and whip until the egg whites are stiff but not dry or until they stand in peaks that lean over slightly. Then beat in the sugar substitute, 1 tablespoon at a time, being careful not to overbeat. Beat in the vanilla. Spread the mixture in the pie shell and bake for 10 to 15 minutes until the meringue is slightly browned on top.

Good for A, B, and C dieters.

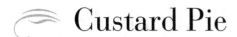

Custard Pie

MAKES ONE 9-INCH PIE.

This is another standard recipe that is complemented by whatever ingredient you decide to add for fun, flavor, and ingenuity. Custard pies must stay and be served well chilled. This recipe is meant to be poured directly into the hot pie crust. Do not let the pie crust cool before putting the custard into it and returning the crust to the oven.

3 eggs or 6 egg yolks
½ cup lo-han or Splenda
¼ teaspoon salt
2 cups heavy cream
1 teaspoon real vanilla extract
1 Macadamia Nut Crumb Crust (see recipe, page 262)

Preheat the oven to 325°F.

In a medium-size mixing bowl, beat the eggs slightly, then add the remaining ingredients and stir well. When the custard is mixed and the pie shell is ready, pour the custard into the hot pie shell and bake for about 30 minutes or until the custard is firm.

Good for A, B, and C dieters.

Chocolate Custard Pie

MAKES ONE 9-INCH PIE.

2 ounces unsweetened dark chocolate

Follow the previous recipe to make the custard filling, then melt the chocolate into the custard mixture. Bake as described in the previous recipe.

Good for A, B, and C dieters.

Pecan Custard Pie

MAKES ONE 9-INCH PIE.

1 teaspoon pecan extract
½ cup pecans, crushed
1 Macadamia Nut Crumb Crust (see recipe, page 262)

Follow the basic Custard Pie recipe to make the custard filling, then stir the pecan extract into the custard. Pour the custard filling into the pie shell, then sprinkle the crushed pecans evenly over it and bake as described in the Custard Pie recipe.

Good for A, B, and C dieters.

Coconut Custard Pie

MAKES ONE 9-INCH PIE.

This is a variation on the traditional pie filling, and it is absolutely delicious.

1 cup flaked unsweetened coconut, plus another ¼ cup
Macadamia nut oil spray
1 Macadamia Nut Crumb Crust (see recipe, page 262)

Follow the Basic Custard Pie recipe to make the custard filling, then blend 1 cup of the untoasted coconut flakes into the heated custard and bake it as described in the Custard Pie recipe. While the pie is baking, in a medium skillet that has been sprayed with macadamia nut oil, allow the oil to get hot and then add the remaining ¼ cup of coconut flakes and cook until they are toasted. Sprinkle the toasted coconut onto the custard pie when it's almost finished baking, with about 2 minutes remaining.

Good for A, B, and C dieters.

Lemon Custard Pie

MAKES ONE 9-INCH PIE.

½ cup lemon juice, freshly squeezed
1 teaspoon lemon zest
1 Macadamia Nut Crumb Crust (see recipe, page 262)

Add the lemon juice to the mixture, then follow the basic Custard Pie recipe exactly until the custard is poured into the shell. At that time, sprinkle the zest throughout, and bake the pie as described in the Custard Pie recipe.

Good for A, B, and C dieters.

Key Lime Custard Pie

MAKES ONE 9-INCH PIE.

½ cup key lime juice, freshly squeezed or bottled
1 teaspoon zest
1 Macadamia Nut Crumb Crust (see recipe, page 262)

This is made exactly as described in the Lemon Custard Pie recipe, except for the substitution of the lime juice.

Good for A, B, and C dieters.

Strawberry or Raspberry Custard Pie

MAKES ONE 9-INCH PIE.

¼ cup strawberries or raspberries, pureed
Additional fruit for garnish
1 Macadamia Nut Crumb Crust (see recipe, page 262)

Follow the basic Custard Pie recipe to make the custard filling, then add the pureed fruit to the custard. Pour the mixture into the pie shell and bake as described in the Custard Pie recipe. When you remove this pie from the oven, place halved strawberries or whole raspberries around the edge of the pie.

Good for A, B, and C dieters.

Chocolate Cream Pie

SERVES 10.

This is a perfect filling for that pie crust and a must for all chocolate lovers out there. It is so rich and creamy you would never know it's healthy.

¾ cup heavy cream
½ cup crème fraîche
4 ounces unsweetened chocolate, chopped in food processor
½ cup Xylitol
Chocolate Whipped Cream (see recipe, page 255)
1 Macadamia Nut Crumb Crust (see recipe, page 262)

Place all the ingredients into the top of a double boiler over hot water. Whisk until well blended and the mixture begins to form small bubbles along the outside rim. Remove the mixture from the heat, and continue whisking until the chocolate becomes shiny and begins to cool. Set it aside to cool, and make the topping. Spoon the cooled filling into a prebaked pie shell. Top with Chocolate Whipped Cream. Serve immediately or refrigerate.

Good for B and C dieters.

Frozen Chocolate Mud Pie

Make Chocolate Cream Pie (page 267) and Chocolate Whipped Cream Topping (page 255) and instead of placing one on top of the other, use a rubber spatula to fold the chocolate filling and chocolate whipped cream topping together. Blend well without breaking down the whipped cream. Spoon into a pie shell, wrap well with plastic wrap, and freeze. Slice the pie when it is frozen. This is a great way to eat one small piece at a time. I like to make it this way and then cut it into individual serving sizes. This way, when I'm hankering for a chocolate fix, it's already portioned out and I don't have to worry about eating too much at once.

Good for B and C dieters.

Chocolate Decadence Ice Cream

MAKES SIX ½-CUP SERVINGS.

This is by far one of the best chocolate ice creams I have ever tasted. You would never know it wasn't Häagen-Dazs—my secret addiction that I allow myself to have twice a year.

2 cups heavy cream
¾ cup Xylitol
½ cup cocoa powder, Dutch-processed, unsweetened
¼ teaspoon sea salt

Whisk together all the ingredients in a mixing bowl. Pour into an ice cream maker or a tray and freeze.

Good for A, B, and C dieters.

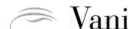 # Vanilla Decadence Ice Cream

Follow the recipe for Chocolate Decadence Ice Cream (page 269), but leave out the cocoa powder. In a mini food processor or blender, grind up 1 vanilla bean and add it to the mixture before putting it into the ice cream maker. This will be the richest vanilla ice cream you've ever tasted.

Good for A, B, and C dieters.

Crème aux Fraises

SERVES 8–10.

This is nothing more than strawberries and cream, but with a twist—French style. The recipe comes from Lyon, France. Jeff ate this in a little café and asked the waiter for the recipe. The waiter was reluctant to give it to him, but Jeff is a persistent fellow, so he went back and asked the chef. The chef was thrilled that a chef from America wanted his simple recipe, and now we are sharing it with you. This is a wonderful late-spring-to-summer recipe, when the fruit is at its ripest.

3 pints fresh strawberries, washed and stemmed
1 tablespoon kirsch (cherry liqueur)
½ cup Splenda or lo-han
1½ cups heavy cream, very cold
Fresh mint for garnish

Put a mixing bowl and beaters from an electric mixer in the refrigerator to chill. Puree the strawberries in a blender or food processor, then strain out the seeds by pressing the berries through a large, fine-meshed sieve. Discard the seeds. Add the kirsch and sweetener to the seedless strawberry puree, stirring to dissolve. Remove the bowl and beaters from the refrigerator and whip the cream until it's stiff. Carefully fold the cream into the pureed strawberries. Transfer to a glass or crystal bowl, cover with plastic wrap, and refrigerate until ready to serve. Just before serving, garnish with mint.

Good for A, B, and C dieters.

Baked Apple with Walnuts

SERVES 6–12.

Sticking to our theme of fresh, local, and seasonal delights, in the fall this combination can't be beat. Try to get large, tart red apples, but whatever grows best in your part of the world will do just fine.

6 large baking apples
½ cup walnuts, chopped
1 packet stevia
¼ cup water
¼ teaspoon nutmeg, freshly grated
¼ teaspoon ground cinnamon
1 tablespoon butter

Preheat the oven to 350°F.

Core the apples and place them into a 6- × 10-inch baking dish. Fill the apples with the walnuts. In a saucepan, combine the stevia, water, spices, and butter. Bring to a boil. Drizzle the hot syrup onto the apples, then bake them uncovered for about 1 hour.

Good for B and C dieters; one-half serving is good for A dieters.

Applesauce

This is fun, easy, and great in the fall months. I recommend that you use this recipe as an excuse to go apple picking at your nearest farm. Even if the apples aren't organic, you will at least get apples that are local and seasonal to your part of the country. This makes for a great family outing and teaches the kids about seasonal harvesting. This dish can be made in great quantities and stored in the refrigerator for about a week, and it can be added to other dishes to make them more appealing for fussy eaters. It's also a great recipe for the new mom. Jeff recommends using red apples such as Gala or whatever grows in your neck of the woods.

4 red apples
2 tablespoons lemon juice, freshly squeezed
½ teaspoon ground cinnamon

Peel and core the apples and cut them into small pieces. Put the apple pieces and lemon juice into a food processor. Blend until the mixture is smooth. Put this mixture into a medium saucepan and bring to a simmer over medium heat. Stir constantly for about 10 minutes until it is reduced by one quarter. Stir in the cinnamon. Serve the applesauce warm or cold.

Good for A, B, and C dieters.

Coconutty Fruit Kabobs

SERVES 8.

The most difficult part of this recipe is finding the 8-inch skewers. Then you can use whatever fruit you have around the house or whatever happens to be fresh and seasonal at the market that day. Of course, we emphasize low-glycemic fruits. You can refer to the pyramids at the beginning of this book to make sure you get the healthiest fruits.

1 pear
1 apricot
20 red and green seedless grapes
½ honeydew melon
1 green apple, peeled, cored, and cut into small chunks
1 cup yogurt, plain, sugar-free
½ cup coconut, sugar-free, dried, shredded
8 8-inch skewers

Cut all the fruit into bite-size pieces.

Create your own kabobs by threading the pieces of fruit onto the skewers. Add as much or as little of whatever fruit you want. Do this until the skewer is almost full. Leave enough room to hold on to the dull end.

Put the yogurt on one plate and the coconut on another plate. Roll each kabob in the yogurt, then the coconut. Repeat these steps with each kabob until all are coconut coated. Eat right away or freeze for about 5 minutes until the yogurt and coconut are fully set.

Good for B and C dieters.

Peach Crush

This is a great way to enjoy peaches on a hot summer day. It also may tempt toddlers and other people who don't eat fruit to enjoy some healthful antioxidants. I'm a big believer in disguising the taste of healthy food in a form that people think is unhealthy—it really works.

1 cup heavy cream
½ cup water
2 cups fresh peaches, sliced

Pour the cream and water into an ice cube tray and freeze until solid. Pop the frozen cubes out of the tray and put them into the blender, along with the peaches. Blend at high speed until creamy and smooth. Pour the peach crush into glasses and serve.

A variation on this recipe is to put the cream, water, and peaches into a blender or a food processor and blend, then pour it into ice pop molds, inserting the sticks when the pops are partly frozen. This is a healthy ice pop, and it tastes great. This recipe can be used with any fruit that you or that finicky person may enjoy. I find it to be a great end to a summer barbecue, without the fanciness of a proper dessert. All the kids at a party love it, and it turns adults into kids again.

Good for A, B, and C dieters.

Hamptons Diet Desserts   275

Strawberry Cantaloupe Crush

SERVES 4.

This is just like the peach crush, but we replaced the peaches with strawberries and cantaloupe. As with many of the recipes in this book, use your imagination.

1 cup heavy cream
½ cup water
1 cup fresh strawberries
1 cup cantaloupe

Pour the cream and water into an ice cube tray and freeze until solid. Pop the frozen cubes out of the tray and put them into the blender, along with the strawberries and cantaloupe.

Blend at high speed until creamy and smooth. Pour the strawberry and cantaloupe crush into glasses and serve.

Again, the same variation as described in the previous recipe can turn these into fun ice pops.

Good for A, B, and C dieters.

Gluten- and Grain-Free Cookies

The next four recipes are made without grains of any kind and so they are perfect for people who suffer from a gluten sensitivity. Each of these recipes behaves a little differently because the nuts have varying textures, densities, and fat contents. Since these cookies are made without flour, follow the directions very carefully.

Almond Cookies

MAKES 16 COOKIES.

These cookies are unbelievably delicious and rich. For this reason, two of them are plenty and are the recommended serving size. Try freezing the cookies that you aren't going to eat on the day that you make them, because they are difficult to resist.

¼ cup unsalted almonds, ground in food processor
    (or get almond flour at specialty stores or online).
    Measure almonds after grinding.
¼ cup natural, smooth almond butter
⅓ cup cream cheese, room temperature
1 teaspoon almond extract
½ teaspoon vanilla extract
2 tablespoons Xylitol
2 tablespoons whey protein (vanilla bean flavor)
½ teaspoon baking powder
½ tablespoon almonds, thinly sliced (16 slices)

Preheat the oven to 375°F.

Put all the ingredients except the sliced almond into the bowl of an electric mixer in the order listed. Beat at a medium speed until well blended.

Dip your fingers in cold water and roll the dough into walnut-sized balls. Carefully place the balls on a parchment paper–lined cookie sheet. Place a slivered almond in the center of each cookie. Bake for 10 minutes. Remove to a cooling rack and allow to cool completely before you eat them.

Good for A, B, and C dieters.

conut Pecan Cookies

16 COOKIES.

⅓ cup unsalted pecans, ground in a food processor.
   Measure pecans after grinding.
⅓ cup coconut, unsweetened, shredded
⅓ cup cream cheese, room temperature
1 teaspoon vanilla extract
2 tablespoons Xylitol
1 tablespoon whey protein (vanilla bean flavor)
½ teaspoon baking powder
2 tablespoons pecans (16 halves)

Preheat the oven to 375°F.

Put all the ingredients except the pecan halves into the bowl of an electric mixer in the order listed. Beat at a medium speed until well blended.

Wet your fingers with cold water. Roll the mixture into walnut-sized balls and place them on a parchment paper–lined cookie sheet. Press a pecan half into the center of each cookie. Bake for 10 minutes. Remove to a rack and allow to cool before you eat them.

Good for A, B, and C dieters.

Walnut Chocolate Chip Cookies

MAKES 16 COOKIES.

¼ cup unsalted walnuts, ground in food processor.
    Measure walnuts after grinding.

¼ cup unsweetened cocoa powder

¼ cup cream cheese, room temperature

1 teaspoon vanilla extract

2 tablespoons Xylitol

1 tablespoon whey protein (vanilla bean flavor)

½ teaspoon baking powder

16 unsweetened chocolate chips or 2 tablespoons walnuts
    (16 walnut halves)

Preheat the oven to 375°F.

Put all the ingredients except the chocolate chips or walnut halves into the bowl of an electric mixer in the order listed. Beat at a medium speed until well blended.

Roll the mixture into walnut-sized balls and place them on a parchment paper–lined cookie sheet. Gently press a chocolate chip or walnut half into the center of each cookie. Bake for 10 minutes. Remove to a rack and allow to cool before you eat them.

Good for A, B, and C dieters.

Peanut Butter Cookies

MAKES 16 COOKIES.

¼ cup unsalted peanuts, ground in food processor.
 Measure peanuts after grinding.
¼ cup smooth, natural peanut butter (without added sugar)
⅓ cup cream cheese, room temperature
1 teaspoon vanilla extract
2 tablespoons Xylitol
1 tablespoon whey protein (vanilla bean flavor)
½ teaspoon baking powder
2 teaspoons peanuts (16 peanut halves)

Preheat the oven to 375°F.

Put all the ingredients except the peanut halves into the bowl of an electric mixer in the order listed. Beat at a medium speed until well blended.

Roll the mixture into walnut-sized balls and place them on a parchment paper–lined cookie sheet. Gently press half a peanut into the center of each cookie. Bake for 10 minutes. Remove to a rack and allow to cool before you eat them.

Good for A, B, and C dieters.

Resource Guide and Contact Information

There are many places to get exquisite foods, and I recommend that you use the Internet to find them. Who knows? Many of them may be in your neighborhood. Another trick that works quite well for my patients is to ask their local butcher, grocery store, and so on, to carry things for them. The store owner or the manager is often willing to make special orders for you, especially if he or she knows you would be willing to pay a little extra for the service.

Fish

This is such a controversial topic right now, with the combined problems of mercury toxicity, overfishing, and unhealthy farming practices, that I felt it was necessary to mention the one place where I get all of my fish when I cook at home. The name of the company is Vital Choice, and it can be reached at www.vitalchoice.com. Its product is from Alaska and Canada, and each batch is tested for mercury. The company also practices protective catching of the fish to ensure that the stock does not get depleted. The fish are a little more expensive but are absolutely the best I have ever eaten.

Salt

I know this may seem like an odd thing to recommend, but it really is an important part of most people's diet and a source of contamination if you aren't using the right brand. The brand I highly recommend is RealSalt™. This salt is not bleached, kiln dried, heated, or altered with chemicals or pollutants. It also has a full complement of trace minerals, including calcium, potassium, sulfur, magnesium, iron, phosphorus, iodine, manganese, copper, and zinc. RealSalt comes from an ancient sea bed in Utah. This salt is from an ocean that existed millions of years before pollution contaminated our planet. During the time that dinosaurs roamed the earth, volcanoes erupted near this sea bed, sealing the salt with layers of volcanic ash so that no modern pollutants have touched it either. It has an amazing flavor and, like MacNut Oil, adds an indescribable hint of goodness to any dish. You can get RealSalt at many fine food stores, by calling 1-800-367-7258, or at www.realsalt.com.

Sustainable Agriculture

Since the Hamptons Diet is all about getting back to nature and eating foods that are close to nature, without harming the land, I have composed a short list of local farms in the New York City area that sell properly raised and fed beef, chicken, turkey, pork, duck, lamb, and eggs. These are

1.   Hawthorne Valley Farm, Ghent, New York
2.   DiPaola Turkeys, Trenton, New Jersey
3.   Flying Pigs Farm, Shushan, New York
4.   Quattro's Game Farm, Pleasant Valley, New York

I now have an online store so that my Hamptonites can find out where to get some of the highest-quality foods and nutritional supplements that are compatible with the Hamptons Diet. You can sign up for my newsletter, *The Hamptonite*; there is also an online blog (which I visit from time to time) so that dieters can help each other out. I encourage each of you to visit www.hamptonsdietmarketplace.com.

Macadamia Nut Oil

Since I first wrote *The Hamptons Diet*, there has been an incredible public response to macadamia nut oil. In fact, there has been such a rush on the oil that a world shortage has occurred for the foreseeable future. I have therefore had to expand my base of oils and have found excellent sources in Kenya and South Africa. It is not essential to have 100 percent Australian oil anymore. Many companies are now trying to sell macadamia nut oil. Like most things, however, only a few are reputable.

MacNut Oil is the gold standard on which all other macadamia nut oils should be based. The company can be easily contacted through www .macnutoil.com or by calling 1-866-4MACNUT. That site has a great free newsletter that you can sign up for, and you can find the store nearest you that sells the oil or order it directly and have it shipped right to your door. Whole Foods and many other natural markets now carry this brand.

Contact the Authors

Of course, if you need or want to get in contact with me, I will always love to hear from you. I can be reached at my Web site: www.hamptonsdiet.com. My current office address is

274 Madison Avenue, Suite 402

New York, NY 10016

212-779-2944

212-779-2941 (fax)

If there are any changes to my contact information, I will post them on the office Web site: www.piimdocs.com.

Jeff Harter can be reached at www.spanishcuisineconsultant.com.

Shallots, Green Beans with, 184
Shellfish Cocktail, 79
Shiitake Mushrooms, in Simmered
    Shrimp with Scallions, 83
shrimp
    Diablo, 124
    Simmered, with Shiitake Mushrooms
        and Scallions, 83
    Steamed, and New Zealand Cockles,
        123
    Stuffed Mushrooms, 219
Siciliana, 232
side dishes
    about, 151–52
    recipes, 153–94. *See also individual
        names of dishes*
Simmered Shrimp with Shiitake Mush-
    rooms and Scallions, 83
Sleepy Hollow Ultimate Chicken Salad
    Sandwich, 71
Snow Pea Salad, 162–63
Sonoran Ultimate Chicken Salad Sand-
    wich, 72
soups
    Almond, Chilled, with Oven-Roasted
        Figs and Coconut Mascarpone,
        251–52
    Broccoli Cheese, 104
    Creamy Chickpea and Farro Soup,
        106–7
    Fish Chowder, Main Beach, 80
    Gazpacho Andalucia, 99
    Lentil, 97–98
    Mama Pescatore Lentil, 97–98
    Quick and Easy Chicken Rice, 100
    Red Pepper, 217
    Roasted Tomato and Onion Soup with
        Fresh Herbs, 105
    Spinach Parmesan, 68
    Summer Squash, 96
Sour Cream, with Braised Brussels
    Sprouts and Bacon, 149
Southampton Crab Cakes, 82
Southampton Omelet, 45
Southampton Vinaigrette, 170

Spaghetti Squash, 190
Spanish Blue Cheese, Endive with, 216
Spareribs, Barbecued, 94
spices. *See individual names of spices*
Spicy Almonds, 223
Spicy Buffalo Meatballs in Mushroom
    Cream Sauce, 135
Spicy Eye Round, 108–9
Spicy Plum Island Sauce, 202
Spicy Sauce, 108–9
spinach
    and Cheese, Pine Nut Stuffing,
        127–28
    and Parmesan Soup, 68
    Salmon with, 119–20
Springs Picante Dip, 205
squash
    Soup, Summer, 96
    Spaghetti, 190
steak
    Chicken-Fried Steak Fingers, 200
    Grilled Hanger Steak, 147
Steamed Shrimp and New Zealand
    Cockles, 123
strawberries
    and Cantaloupe Crush, 275
    with Crème aux Fraises, 271
    in Custard Pie, 266
Stuffed Pimientos, 235
Stuffed Pork Chops with Spinach,
    Cheese, and Pine Nuts, 127–28
Stuffing, Couscous, 175
Summer Squash Soup, 96
Summer Vegetable Medley, 183
Sweet Potatoes, Whipped, Southern
    Style, 191
Swiss Chard Rounds, 188–89
Swiss Crackers, 227

Tamari Macadamia Dressing, 77–78
Tangy Cucumber (Zucchini) and Tuna
    Wrap, 81
Teriyaki, Grilled Halibut with, 146
Thyme, in Double Pork Chop with
    Lemon, 130

294   *Recipe Index*

INDEX

shopping for, 25–30
food co-ops (cooperatives), 25
food processors, mini, 19
food pyramids, 6–7
  carbohydrate (grain), 9
  carbohydrate (vegetable), 8
  fats/oils, 10–11
  fruit, 9–10
  protein, 7–8
free radicals, 30
free range poultry, 27–28
freezing, of foods, 20
fruit, 11
  brushes for, 21
  food pyramid, 9–10
  healthy choices for, 24–25
  shopping for, 25–33
  storage of, 20
  See also sweeteners

Gare, Fran, 211
gluten, 277
grains, 11
  "whole grain," defined, 28
  "whole wheat," defined, 26
greenmarkets, 24–25
grilling, 139
grocery stores, 25
guar gum, 61

Hamptons, 24
Hamptons Diet, 5–6
  A, B, C plans, 6
  food pyramids for, 6–11
  top ten rules of, 12–13
Hamptons Diet, The (Pescatore), 1, 2
Hamptons Diet Cookbook, The (Pescatore, Harter), 3–4
hand-held immersion blenders, 19
Harter, Edna, 41
Harter, Jeff, 2–4, 30
hazelnut oil, 32, 33
herbs, 26
hormone-free foods, 28
Hurt, Alison Becker, 2, 201

hydrogenated oils, 31

kitchen set-up, 15–16
  appliances, 18–19
  baking implements, 17
  cutting boards, 17–18
  healthy ingredients and, 23–25
  miscellaneous items for, 20–23
  mixing bowls, measuring cups, storage, 20
  pots, pans, 16–17
  utensils, 19

labels on foods, 26–29
lauric acid, 259
leftovers, 20
legumes, 11
Lo-Han fruit, 248

macadamia nut oil, 5, 12
  fats in, 32
  MacNut Oil, 23
maltitol, 249
mandolins, for food preparation, 21
margarine, 33
measuring cups, 20
meat thermometers, 21
Mediterranean diet, 1–2, 5
mini-food processors, 19
mixing bowls, 20
monounsaturated fats, 12, 31

"natural" foods, defined, 28
nitrates/nitrites, 29
non-GMO (genetically modified) foods, 27
"no sugar added," defined, 28, 250
Nutrasweet, 249–50
nuts, 11

oils, 12
  cooking oil comparison, 32
  food pyramid for, 10–11
  healthy choices for, 30–33
  smoke point of, 30–31